Pernicious Anaemia:
the forgotten disease

the causes and consequences
of
vitamin B_{12} deficiency

'All shall be well, and all shall be well, and all manner of thing shall be well.'

Julian of Norwich

Pernicious Anaemia: the forgotten disease

the causes and consequences of vitamin B_{12} deficiency

By
Martyn Hooper

Foreword by
Professor A David Smith and Professor Helga Refsum

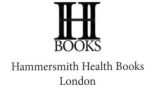

Hammersmith Health Books
London

First published in 2012 by Hammersmith Health Books – an imprint of
Hammersmith Books Limited
14 Greville Street, London EC1N 8SB, UK
www.hammersmithbooks.co.uk

British Library Cataloguing in Publication Data: A CIP record of this
book is available from the British Library.

Print ISBN 978-1-78161-004-6
Ebook ISBN 978-1-78161-005-3
Commissioning editor: Georgina Bentliff
Designed and typeset by: Julie Bennett
Index: Dr Laurence Errington
Production: Helen Whitehorn, Pathmedia
Printed and bound by TJ International Ltd
Cover image: The Heavy Burden by Honore Daumier, reproduced by
permission of the National Museum of Wales

Contents

Acknowledgements

I have received a great deal of help and support in researching and writing this book, not only in the information I have been given, but also in the way some complex science was explained to me in language that I, as a non-scientist, could understand. The following people all deserve to be congratulated, not only for helping me to write this book, but also for their patience and for making allowance for my limited scientific knowledge.

Thanks to:

- Dr Fiona Smith-Porter for her brutal assassination of chapter 5 and for helping to give a GP's perspective of the diagnostic procedure that was included in the re-write;
- Dr Joe Chandy, Dr Hugo Minney and the members of the B_{12} D group;
- Mr Dick Ellis of the University Hospital of Wales, Cardiff, for his help in revising chapter 2;
- Professor David Smith and Professor Helga Refsum from Oxford University for their enthusiastic support for this project and for taking the time to explain patiently to someone who has no knowledge of science that there is indeed a difference between a pg/ml and pmol/ml;
- The members of the Pernicious Anaemia Society for sending me their personal stories of late or wrong diagnosis – sadly, I was able to use only a few due to the book's word limit;

Acknowledgements

- Sally Pacholok and Jeffery Stuart for their tireless work in raising awareness of the consequences of B_{12} deficiency and their thoroughly convincing explanation of why the current threshold level for determining B_{12} deficiency is far too low;
- Pat Kornic and her team of Moderators who do such a good job in helping people to understand their condition, including myself;
- Andrea McArthur for her relentless efforts to raise awareness of the problems with diagnosing and treating pernicious anaemia among politicians and medical professionals;
- Dr Zeena Nackerdien for her advice, guidance and suggestions;
- Jon Patchet and his team at Tastic Multimedia without whose help and support the Pernicious Anaemia Society would not exist;
- Mr Ian McLean of San Francisco for his remarkable research which uncovered several items in this book;
- Rhianna Eluned Carter for reading through the very first draft of chapter 2 and giving a science teacher's viewpoint regarding readability;
- All of the volunteers who give so freely of their time to the Pernicious Anaemia Society and, in particular, Mr Kenneth Davies and Miss Rasa Cibulskyte, whose work constructing the charts and organising the pictures was invaluable;
- Georgina Bentliff of Hammersmith Health Books for her encouragement and patience;
- and finally to my wife for letting me take over the dining table for the last six months, for not moaning about the chaotic mess of papers and books and for her continued support and understanding.

Hopefully this book will be the catalyst that will lead to a thorough review of the way in which pernicious anaemia in particular, and B_{12} deficiency in general, are diagnosed and treated. That can only be a good thing.

Preface

When I was eventually diagnosed with vitamin B_{12} deficiency caused by pernicious anaemia in May 2002, my first reaction was to look for an easy to understand explanation of the condition. To my dismay there was no such material available. For a year I struggled to try to understand what caused the problem and, slowly, I began to comprehend the basics of the disease.

In mid-October 2004, I was forced to take early retirement from my career and decided to use my time to ensure that anyone who was diagnosed with vitamin B_{12} deficiency and/or pernicious anaemia would be able to access information about the disease and, perhaps, interact with other sufferers. Now this is important; all that I set out to do was to provide an easy to understand information leaflet that would explain in lay terms just what pernicious anaemia was. At the time I was diagnosed, Wikipedia was in its infancy and didn't produce any result for 'pernicious anaemia', while more general internet searching for the term produced only vague results involving a handful of documents and articles that were written by and for medical professionals. They might have been in another language.

I knew that I would need some sort of website and so I contacted, via email, around 25 web-designers, whose details I had found after searching online, asking if they would consider helping out a small charity that was just forming – although I had no intention at this time of forming a charity; it just seemed more likely that I might be successful if I said that. I was, as you can see, not only cheeky but also extremely naïve about how the third (or charity) sector works. I had a few apologetic replies and then, in November 2004, I received a reply from a web-designer who offered to design, for free, a website with an online forum that would let other sufferers gain information about the condition from other people with pernicious anaemia. It turned out that the designer, Jon Patchet of Tastic Multimedia, was just starting out on his own and had made the decision that he would sponsor a charity from the very beginning of his business. I didn't know what a 'forum' was and after a short telephone call with Jon I set out to visit him in North Wales. I remember that it began snowing over the Brecon Beacons, but I arrived safely and I sat down with Jon and discussed my requirements, and Jon described how an online forum would allow members to interact with each other. I travelled back home the same day and by the time I got home there was a single-page website on the internet.

A few days later the online forum was ready. Within an hour of going 'live', the first forum user had registered and had posted her story. It was remarkably similar to mine – she had gone undiagnosed for years and felt that she was receiving inadequate treatment. Yet she was not from the UK but from the United States. Within two days the number of people on the forum was in double figures and in just over a week there were over one hundred registered users. Some of the users were asking for information, but the majority were taking the opportunity to tell their own stories of misdiagnosis and inadequate treatment regimes. What had started out as a project to inform sufferers of pernicious anaemia about the cause and treatment of the disease had suddenly become a place where users could vent their frustration and anger at the poor standard of diagnosis and treatment.

It became clear that there were serious issues surrounding pernicious anaemia that hadn't been addressed for decades. For the first time, patients with the condition had a medium through which they could not only find out more, but also share their stories of travelling down a very long road before receiving, eventually, a diagnosis and discovering how others dealt with the problem of inadequate treatment. What had started out as an online 'bulletin board' for patients and their families and friends in the UK had quickly transformed into an international seminar that drew attention to the significant problems with the symptoms, diagnosis and treatment of a quite common disease.

The Pernicious Anaemia Society has grown from an online forum into a registered and influential international charity with over six and a half thousand members. It is still growing and its remit is not only to provide information for patients and their families and friends, but also to bring about changes in how sufferers are diagnosed and treated, mainly by raising awareness among medical professionals of the problems faced by members of the Society. To date the charity is still campaigning, with some success, to bring about these changes.

Any case studies used in this book have been written by members of the Pernicious Anaemia Society who have given permission for their stories to be used. These case studies are for illustrative purposes only and, like the results of the Society's online survey that is quoted within the book, substantiate the stories told on the online forum and the telephone calls the Society receives regularly. More sad and bad experiences of patients suffering from pernicious anaemia can be found on the online forum and on the many Facebook pages set up for people not only with pernicious anaemia but also for those suffering from B_{12} deficiency. The reader is advised to visit these pages to understand just how big the problems are for patients getting quickly and accurately diagnosed and treated.

Foreword

You probably think, as do many doctors, that vitamins are 'old hat' and that nowadays everyone in developed countries has a diet that is more than adequate in its vitamin content. How often have you heard people say that 'all you need is a good balanced diet'? Apart from the difficulty in defining a 'good balanced diet', this remark does not take into account two factors: first, we are living much longer, and our nutritional needs change as we age; second, we have different genetic make-ups and some people need extra amounts of some of the vitamins. One of the best examples is the subject of this book: the disease called pernicious anaemia, which is a particular case of extreme vitamin B_{12} deficiency.

Vitamin B_{12} is one of the vitamins that we need in very small amounts, as little as a few micrograms each day. It is made only by certain bacteria and, except for these bacterial sources, it is found just in animal-derived foods. The process whereby we obtain B_{12} from animal-derived foods is complex and, in normal ageing, some aspects of this process may become inefficient and so absorption from the gastrointestinal tract fails and deficiency develops. B_{12}-deficiency, or poor B_{12} status, is common in the elderly with about 20 per cent showing signs of it. But the widely held view that B_{12}-deficiency is found only in the elderly is wrong; it can occur at all stages of life, from the breast-fed infant, to the pregnant woman, to the strict vegetarian.

The consequences of poor B_{12} status have recently been recognised as more far-reaching than originally thought. Pernicious anaemia, caused by loss of gastric parietal cells which are responsible, in part, for the secretion of a protein called Intrinsic Factor that is critical for absorption of vitamin B_{12} in the intestine, can cause a rapidly developing vitamin B_{12} deficiency with very serious consequences for health, as so well described in this book. However, there are many more subtle harmful effects of low vitamin B_{12} status that have been found in people who do not have such an extreme form of B_{12} deficiency, or in the early phases of pernicious anaemia; such people have blood levels that are often considered normal, or 'low-normal'. These effects include an increased risk of, for example, cognitive decline and Alzheimer's disease, rapid shrinkage of the brain over time, depression, stroke, neural tube defects, like spina bifida, and osteoporosis. These newer findings show that we need more research on the functions of vitamin B_{12}. The remarkable story described in this book also shows that we need more research on the treatment of B_{12}-deficiency and on the reasons why different people need very different amounts of B_{12} to relieve their symptoms.

This book is to be warmly welcomed. It is a vivid and very well-written account of a 'hidden chapter' in medicine that ought to be widely known among the public at large, among policy-makers, and among medical professionals. A major reappraisal of how we define, diagnose and treat B_{12}-deficiency is needed, and this book is a trail-blazer for that mission.

A David Smith   FMedSci
Professor Emeritus of Pharmacology
Hon. Associate Director, MRC Anatomical Neuropharmacology Unit,
University of Oxford

Helga Refsum   MD
Professor of Nutrition, University of Oslo
Visiting Professor of Human Nutrition, University of Oxford

Chapter 1

My story

My story starts in September 2001. The previous year I had turned 40 and I was in my 18th year of lecturing in Further Education. I had a very active lifestyle, running a popular National Diploma course for full-time students, and in my spare time hill walking and leading walking expeditions, playing drums in a rock band, teaching drum-kit to exam standards, and playing tennis. I was a Senior Examiner for A-Level Politics and an examiner for the Chartered Institute of Marketing's Professional Qualifications. I was always 'on the go'. Then around late 2001 I started to feel really tired for the first time in my life. I knew what it was like to be tired after three days of hill walking – and that was a nice tired. But this tiredness was more than physical and mental exhaustion. It was a ubiquitous and insidious tiredness that never really went away. I was even tired after a good night's sleep. Like many other people of my age, I put this strange feeling down to my reaching middle age. There were other little indicators that middle age had arrived. I started to forget things, even found concentrating to be more and more difficult, and began to experience breathlessness more and more. 'This is it,' I thought. 'It's all downhill from here.'

I still kept up my hectic lifestyle and one evening I was playing in a band at a local gig. At the end of the set, and in true rock-star fashion, I jumped off the stage onto the dance-floor below. I landed in a pool of what was probably beer and found myself suddenly horizontal about five feet above the floor before suddenly falling hard on my back. It was quite a spectacular piece of cabaret for a finale and the crowd were genuinely pleased to see me get up and laugh off the whole event. There was apparently no damage done.

A few days later my legs went numb overnight. I awoke in the morning and realised that I had no feeling from my toes up to the middle of my thighs. And my feet and knees seemed to be bloated. 'Probably due to the fall,' I thought. 'They'll return to normal soon.'

They didn't. After a month or six weeks of having no feeling in my legs and feet I booked an appointment with a doctor. It was to be the first of a great many. He didn't seem particularly concerned, explaining that it was probably due to the fall but that it was best to let nature do the healing. I agreed and, reassured that everything would soon be back to normal, resumed my busy life.

The tiredness became increasingly difficult to deal with. Even as a child I had managed on the minimum amount of sleep. I remember being told by my friends' mothers not to knock on their doors before nine o'clock, which meant that for three hours in the mornings I had to occupy myself alone. I can remember thinking it quite unremarkable that Mrs Thatcher needed just four hours' sleep per night. And here I was, having to force myself awake every morning. The breathlessness was bizarre as it seemed to require me to yawn and yawn and yawn as well as take deep breaths one after another. Then my concentration took a dive and I started to have 'fogs'. These are quite difficult to explain to somebody who hasn't experienced them, but it is as if there is a 'fog' that prevents you from understanding things clearly; it's as if something is between you and what you are looking at or hearing or saying. These 'fogs' would last a day, or two, or three. Then I would awake one morning and suddenly everything would be clear again.

Chapter 1

By January 2002 my legs had not repaired and I was now starting to stumble and had developed an ungainly gait – I was walking like Herman Munster. This was around the time that I suddenly became aware that I could not tolerate heights and would become very unsteady on my feet when looking up. There was obviously something wrong and one of the doctors at my local surgery sent me to a neurosurgeon for a consultation.

'Well, you had a fall; you got back up – I don't think this is related to the fall,' he said. 'I want you to have an MRI scan to rule out a number of things.' 'What's an MRI scan?' I asked blankly. He explained that MRI stood for 'magnetic resonance imaging', and that it might be able to explain the numbness and unusual gait that I had developed. I went ahead with the scan, which proved that there was 'nothing sinister there'. (I later discovered that he thought I might have cancer of the spinal cord.) Whilst all of this was going on I was still carrying out my normal hectic schedule and discovering new things wrong with me. In Dublin, with a mini-bus full of students, I stopped to ask the way of two Garda who were walking away from me. I went to run after them, but discovered it was impossible. My legs just wouldn't go fast enough and I made quite a spectacle for the unsympathetic students, who genuinely couldn't see the serious side of what might be going on. I laughed off the incident along with them, but inside I knew that my condition was deteriorating.

In the spring of 2002 I started to have personality changes. I became very irritable with students who sought help or clarification about something. And this was the part of my job that I loved the most – helping people. Now I would treat students as an irritant, and my mood swings were being noticed at home, where I was increasingly short with my wife. It was around this time that I would completely forget a conversation I had had the day before, forget where I had parked my car, get confused trying to write sentences and really just wanted to crawl into a dark hole and sleep. One day, as I left a lecture room I couldn't remember what I had talked about for the past hour before going into another lecture to talk about something for another hour – I didn't know what was happening to me. I started to experience the need to cry for no apparent reason. And I began to realise that I must be depressed. Something would have to be done, but time and time again people would listen to my symptoms and laugh it off as being middle-age related. I tried to laugh with them but was starting to get seriously worried.

I didn't mention the severity of my difficulty trying to cope with everyday life to anyone, not even to any doctor. I thought that the depression was of my own making, and that the physical symptoms were all related to the fall. The tiredness, or rather the chronic fatigue, was all due to middle age – a fact confirmed by others that I talked to.

By mid-May I was close to collapse and, when walking to my local surgery for yet another doctor's appointment, I stumbled, fell in the middle of the road and couldn't get up. I know how it feels to be ridiculed and scorned for being drunk in the middle of the day because as I tried to get up onlookers thought that I was completely inebriated. A police officer eventually helped me to my feet and I convinced him that I was not drunk. 'What's wrong with you?' he asked sympathetically. 'I don't know,' I replied.

The police officer and his colleague kindly took me home in their car – the first and last time I have ever been in a police car. I was confused, frustrated, angry and very, very, very tired. After an hour or so I telephoned my sister. She is additionally a Sister in that she is a nursing sister in the community – what used to be called a District Nurse. She immediately drove to my house where I was stumbling around holding onto anything that was solid to help me walk. She could see that I was in some distress. My main concern was that I had not attended the appointment with the doctor. 'This is ridiculous,' she commented. 'I'm taking blood so that we can get to the bottom of this.' At least that's what I seem to remember. This was not a normal fog that I was in – this was a real pea-souper, with no sign of it lifting. I was the most needle-phobic man on the planet. I would wince at even the thought of a needle, but now I didn't care what she did and where she stuck the needle – I was just not interested. I wanted to sleep.

I can't remember much after she took the blood samples. I can't remember what conversation I had with my wife that evening, and I can't remember how I got to work the next day. But I do know that I was in a lecture room the next day because someone from Personnel popped her head around the door and asked me if she could have a word with me. I stepped out of the classroom and she told me that my doctor had been on the 'phone and that I was to telephone him immediately. They had tried to call me at home, but they had my old number. I went to go back into the class, fully intending to talk what must have been drivel until the end of the lesson. She grabbed my arm.

'I think you ought to telephone him now. He seemed quite concerned.' I went into my work-room. There was nobody else in there as the other staff were all teaching. I telephoned the surgery and asked to be put through to this particular doctor.

'Are you okay?' asked the doctor, who was Irish.

'Yeah,' I lied.

'You need to come to the surgery right now. We have a diagnosis,' he said.

'What is it?'

'I'll explain when you get here. Come straight to my room.'

'I'll come now. How long will I be? I have a class at 12.'

'You'll not be doing any teaching for a while,' he replied. 'At least a week, maybe longer.'

I put the telephone down and went to see my Head of School to explain, or rather not explain, what had happened. She reassured me that there was no problem, but I could already see that I was causing headaches and difficulties. I stumbled to the doctor's surgery and went straight to his room as instructed. I can't remember how I felt. I must have been relieved that at last I had a diagnosis. And I must have been worried as to what that diagnosis would be. But everything was just too much to think about, and I was desperate for any help that I could receive. At the back of my mind must have been the knowledge that this was the only doctor in the practice that I hadn't seen before.

'We think it's sub-acute combined degeneration of the spinal cord secondary to pernicious anaemia,' he said.

I was stunned.

'Can you cure it?'

I remember this bit. I was looking straight into the doctor's face. He looked away. He looked down and to his right.

'We can sort you out. We will sort you out. It'll all be sorted.'

'What will happen?'

'You'll have to go into hospital. You'll have to have blood transfusions. We'll get you in today.'

'How long will I be in hospital?'

'We don't know.'

'A day? Two days? Three?'

'We don't know – maybe a lot longer than that.'

'A week?'

'We don't know.'

'But you can cure me?'

'We'll sort you out.'

'How long will it take to cure?'

'Well, you'll be on injections for life.'

'What kind of injections?'

'Vitamin B_{12} injections. You'll need lots in the next month and then every three months for life.'

'What do I do now?'

'You go home and wait for me to telephone you. Make sure that you give your correct number to reception and let me have it right now.'

'Can you write down what my diagnosis is?'

'Sure.' He wrote down the diagnosis on a slither of paper that advertised some medicine and I stumbled out of the room.

I returned home and waited. My sister was on her way to France and I phoned her mobile. I told her the diagnosis. 'Oh, my God,' was the unhelpful response.

'I have to go into hospital for transfusions,' I told her. 'What am I going to do?'

'Well, you just have to be brave,' she replied in her best 'pull yourself together' tone of voice. I am not a hospital brave; I am a hospital wimp.

I was now very, very confused, tired, exhausted, overwhelmed and unsure what I should do. I didn't know how to react. My emotions were completely out of control and I struggled to be logical. The doctor phoned. There was no need after all to go into hospital. 'Just report to the nurse in the morning for the first of your injections.' I went to bed at three o'clock and slept solidly until eight the next day. I tried to explain things to my wife, but this was difficult. Surely my condition couldn't be due to a vitamin – you could buy vitamins on the high street. This had to be more serious than the lack of a vitamin.

I had stuck the piece of paper on which the doctor had written the diagnosis to the fridge using a magnet.

'Why don't you look it up?' my wife said the next morning. I reached for a dictionary. The root cause was *pernicious* anaemia – the sub-acute thing was secondary to that and so I looked up 'pernicious' in the dictionary. I knew it didn't mean anything nice, but when I saw that the dictionary stated it meant not only 'ruinous' and 'destructive' but, more worryingly, 'fatal', I closed the book.

I reported to the nurse an hour later in an even more confused state than before.

'Do many people have pernicious anaemia?' I asked.

'Not many young people like you, and not many males. It's usually elderly ladies that have it.'

'Do they live long?'

'Oh yes – people used to die of it, but now we've got this.' She held up a small bottle with some reassuring red liquid in it.

'Is that the B_{12}?'

'Yup.'

I looked at the floor when she reached for the syringe and needle.

'Now, the secret is to relax.'

I couldn't relax. I felt a dull ache as the liquid entered my right arm muscle.

'Well done,' she said.

I now know that this isn't the easiest of injections to carry out painlessly. I have heard stories of some patients who have not driven for three months because of the pain of the injection. My first injection was pretty straightforward.

'There – see you tomorrow,' said the nurse.

'How many do I need?'

'Ummmmm,' she consulted some form. 'Doc says every day for a week, then weekly for four weeks, and then monthly for three months, then once every three months for life.'

After three days of injections the pins and needles that I had been experiencing for a year in the tips of my fingers disappeared. After a week, the fog started to clear. After a month I felt that I could cope with life for the first time in two years. I felt confident that improvements would continue.

After the last of my monthly injections I was looking forward to three months of not having one. My physical problems had not improved. My legs were still totally numb from my thighs down to my toes. I still couldn't run, my balance was awful and I found it difficult walking down stairs, but mentally I had become more focused and the fog had lifted. I could handle the physical problems and believed the mental issues would eventually fade away.

I believed that the B_{12} injections had cured me. I was wrong. I now know that there is no cure for pernicious anaemia and that

Chapter 1

the injections are just a way of keeping me alive. They contain B_{12} that replaces the B_{12} that I should be producing. They keep me alive, but they don't cure me.

Six weeks after my last monthly injection I started to feel foggy again. The old symptoms returned with a vengeance. I would talk mumbo-jumbo, state facts that were obvious ('The Queen Mother has died,' I told my wife one day. 'I hope she is dead,' she replied, 'they buried her nine months ago.'); the forgetfulness returned. I became irritable and angry. I suffered severe mood swings. I couldn't cope with work. I panicked. It was all going horribly wrong again. I went back to the doctor's and found the GP who had first made the diagnosis had left the practice.

'I need another injection,' I told the senior partner in the surgery. He sat looking at me – looking at me with intensity; looking at me as if he was examining me; looking at me as if he was searching for signs of any unusual mannerisms. After a few seconds considering my request he said in a quiet voice,

'But you don't need one – every three months is the norm.'

'Perhaps for some people, but not for me,' I argued.

He gently shook his head and I thought he started to smile.

'It's all in your head,' he said. 'Would you like some anti-depressants?'

'It's not in my head. I'm going back to how I was.'

'But you have more B_{12} in your blood than I do,' he said.

'Doc, I know I am going back to how I was, and I don't want to go there. I'm sure another injection would stop it,' I pleaded.

'If I do a blood test it will show that you are practically swimming in B_{12},' he said. 'I am only allowed to give you an injection every three months. Lots of patients believe they need more frequent injections, but *we* know that they don't and that they are imagining it all.'

I remember just staring at him with a completely blank expression.

He stared back. After a few seconds he spoke.

'What if we send you to a haematologist – a blood specialist?'

'No problem,' I said.

A few days later I was in the consulting room of a haematologist who took blood and carried out a full physical examination.

'I need more regular injections,' I pleaded, 'and the doctors won't give me more frequent jabs, but I know, I really know, that I need them.'

'Okay,' he said.

I was speechless. Here was a consultant haematologist who knew far more about blood than the average GP and he was listening to me. I breathed a sigh of relief. It was as if a huge weight had been lifted from my shoulders.

'But why won't they prescribe more frequent jabs?' I asked this angel of a man.

'Because for most people an injection every three months is fine, and the guidelines they follow state three-monthly injections are the norm. But we haematologists know that some people need them more often. Maybe about 18% of people with pernicious anaemia need more regular injections even though the amount of B_{12} in their blood is very high. We simply do not know what goes on at cell level and so, because there is no possibility of overdosing on B_{12}, I'll sanction an injection every month.'

I now know that I was lucky in getting monthly injections. I also know that the 18% figure that the haematologist quoted is completely wrong. The true figure is more like 80%. In addition, I now know that the injections of B_{12} used to be given every month in the 1960s and that was changed to every two months in the 1970s and then to every three months in the 1980s.[i] I also now know that some GPs refuse to sanction more frequent injections even when told to

---

e *British National Formulary*[1] 1984 – the main reference source of treat-
r diseases in the UK.

do so by hospital consultants, whether haematologists or not.

The frequency of injections remains the single most common cause of concern and complaint by members of the Pernicious Anaemia Society that I later went on to form.

Back in the GP's surgery I was in front of yet another GP who was reading the consultant's letter.

'I don't want you to see other doctors. Let me monitor this,' he said. 'This is very interesting.' He smiled at me. 'How often do you want them?'

'I don't know – but I know I can't last three months.' I said. 'My sister will give them to me,' I added.

'Well, what if I write you out a prescription and you keep the ampoules in the fridge – then your sister can give them to you whenever you want?'

'Joy,' I thought.

'That sounds a good idea,' I said.

'This is most unusual,' he said in a friendly manner. 'There is a lot of stuff that we don't know about B_{12},' he admitted before adding, 'Be sure to make any future appointments with me.'

At work it was the end of term and end of year. I looked forward to the coming summer months when I would get better and, hopefully, eventually return to normal. I had been on a roller-coaster for the past two years, but now that I had a diagnosis I was hopeful that after a few months all would be well again. The college that I worked for was sympathetic and after informal negotiations it was agreed that for the coming academic year my timetable would be adjusted so that my lectures would all take place in the mornings. I was still getting tired in the afternoons and so, with my new timetable, I would be able to finish my teaching duties at 1.30 pm. My marking and lesson preparations would be completed in the mornings or the weekends. I had no evening classes timetabled. I coped for a year.

During the summer recess of 2003 I went into the college nearly every day of the six-week holiday. I had four days when

I didn't go in. I used to be at my desk at around 8.30 and would leave at around 1.00 pm. I wrote out lesson plans, updated my notes and hand-outs and completed all of my admin. I had managed one year of coping with the demands of modern teaching and I was determined that I would carry on with my career. But coping was what I was doing. I didn't realise it at the time, but I had developed a *coping strategy*. I was still symptomatic, even though I was up to date with my injections. I was lucky. My employers were sympathetic and had made allowances for my condition.

Towards the end of the six-week holiday I was told by a senior manager at the college that other lecturers were complaining that I was able to finish at 1.30 every day and that, from September, I would be expected to follow a normal timetable that would include two postgraduate evening classes. I couldn't argue, but I suspected that the complaints from other lecturers were a fabrication. I knew that going back to a full day timetable with evening classes would be difficult, but I resigned myself to it.

I was in for a nasty shock. The hectic first week of induction activities was bad enough, but when the work routine began in earnest I started to make stupid mistakes. Modern teaching in Further Education involves more than just lesson preparation and lectures. As a Course Tutor I was expected to perform a host of other duties, including helping students complete university applications, organising personal tutorials, holding team meetings, recording team meetings, preparing an on-going course report and quality control paperwork, plus a great many other associated administrative tasks that I had to do. This was all part of a Further Education teacher's job and it was a relentless round of administration and mentoring with some very demanding students. It was hard enough when I was well, but now I was really struggling. And along with all this I was teaching two evenings a week on a postgraduate MBA programme.

I was floundering and, after one particularly demanding day

and evening, realised that I could no longer cope. I was disciplined informally for my reaction to a particularly unsavoury case of bullying (yes, it does happen at college level) and made up my mind that, because of my condition, I would no longer be able to do the job I loved and I would have to stop teaching.

I resolved to leave and the feeling of relief that I would no longer have to fight to complete what once seemed mere menial tasks is still with me. Looking back I really don't know how I managed to perform my duties for the two years before diagnosis and the year that followed. It makes me shudder to think of it now. Whenever I feel sorry for myself I remind myself of the alternative lifestyle that I struggled to manage.

I have since discovered that my experience was very similar to thousands and thousands of other people's and that, even now, hundreds of other people are going through the same ordeal of trying to get diagnosed quickly and treated adequately. Read the 'My Story' section of the Pernicious Anaemia Society's online forum and you will soon realise that, as Sally Pacholok and Jeffrey Stuart say in their book *Could it be B_{12}?*[2] there is an 'epidemic of misdiagnosis' relating to B_{12} deficiency in general, and pernicious anaemia in particular.

Chapters 4 to 8 address the three main problem areas surrounding pernicious anaemia – namely, the symptoms, the diagnosis and the treatment of the condition. But before that, we need to understand fully just what pernicious anaemia and vitamin B_{12} deficiency are and how the problem comes about.

References

1   *British National Formulary*, London, UK; Royal Pharmaceutical Society & British Medical Association. (Two new editions each year.)
2   Pacholok S, Stuart JS. *Could it be B_{12}? – An Epidemic of Misdiagnosis.* 2nd ed. Fresno, California USA: Quill Driver Books; 2011.

Vitamin B$_{12}$ and psychosis (1)

Psychosis is a general medical term used to describe patients who have lost touch with reality. In the UK, the worst cases will be detained under section 3 of the Mental Health Act 1983 for their own safety.

One of the established causes of psychosis is vitamin B$_{12}$ deficiency. Despite this, Richard J Hart, Jr., MD and Paul R McCurdy, MD had this to say in the *Archives of Internal Medicine* in 1971:

> *'Vitamin B$_{12}$ deficiency may present with a psychosis which is curable if treated promptly. Although this fact is not new and is described in various textbooks, it seems that it is often forgotten, which results in prolonged suffering from irreversible brain damage.'*

Homeopathic doctors such as Jonathan Prousky, Professor of the Canadian College of Naturopathic Medicine, are aware of the use of B$_{12}$ to treat psychiatric illnesses. Here's what he had to say in the *Journal of Orthomolecular Medicine* in 2010:

> *'Vitamin B$_{12}$ (cobalamin) ranks among the most useful, safe, and effective orthomolecules when treating a diverse array of neuropsychiatric conditions. However, most clinicians do not consider vitamin B$_{12}$ important unless the serum level is below laboratory reference ranges.'*

Mood changes and behavioural problems are common symptoms of pernicious anaemia, as we will see, and these often lead to family and work-place problems. Because the vitamin is so cheap and safe it is a wonder that patients with mild to severe psychiatric problems aren't given B$_{12}$ routinely when suspected of having a mental illness.

Chapter 2

Blood, vitamins and B$_{12}$

Vitamin B$_{12}$ is not just very important for good health – it's essential. If a person is deficient in this often overlooked vitamin for long enough, then he or she will at best feel continually tired and suffer from breathing problems, and at worst will develop severe and irreversible nerve damage, leaving him/her with mild to severe balance problems and difficulties with walking. Left untreated, the patient will die a slow drawn-out death. And on that happy note, we will begin our journey towards understanding the nature of B$_{12}$ and what it does.

We will have to begin by understanding a little about blood – and I mean just a little. To understand fully this truly amazing substance would take many years in medical school, with a similar period of postgraduate study; and even then you wouldn't know everything there is to know about blood, but you'd be getting pretty close.

The word 'blood', like no other medical term, has worked its way not only into our literature but lies at the heart (sorry) of most cultures. Christians drink 'the blood of Christ' at mass. Jehovah's Witnesses refuse to eat blood or receive transfusions, based on writings in the scriptures. Blood was, and may still be, used in pagan festivals. Both Islam and Judaism forbid the consumption of blood. In Japanese and Chinese cultures, a bleeding nose is taken as a sign of sexual arousal whilst Australian Aborigines used blood to paint their naked bodies during ceremonies. Then there are the vampires of Eastern Europe, after whom vampire bats (from the New World) were named, and the more recent use of the word falsely to describe the use of blood in rituals – blood libel. And if you think the word is complicated, stay with me and you'll never look at a drop of blood in the same way again.

To understand pernicious anaemia we have first to understand what blood is. The following relates mainly to vertebrates (that's animals with a spine) and I promise I'm not making any of this up.

A short note on blood

Blood, as far as medical professionals are concerned, is technically tissue – just like skin. It is composed of blood cells and plasma. Plasma accounts for around 55% of blood fluid, and is about 92% water. Plasma contains all kinds of interesting stuff, including hormones, mineral ions, glucose and carbon dioxide . Carbon dioxide is the waste product of human metabolism. Blood plasma, without any blood cells, is straw coloured. Blood cells make up the other 45% of blood volume. There are two types of blood cells in blood - red blood cells (RBCs) that make up 44.3% of whole blood and white blood cells that constitute 0.7% of total blood. So, whole blood is made up of:

- 55% plasma
- 44.3% red blood cells
- 0.7% white blood cells, including platelets, which are responsible for blood clotting.

One microlitre of blood (that is one millionth of a litre – a very small amount in any language) will contain:

- 4.7-6.1 million (in men), or 4.2-5.4 million (in women) red blood cells – more scientifically known as 'erythrocytes'; the proportion of blood occupied by red blood cells is referred to as the 'haematocrit'.

- 4,000–11,000 white blood cells, or 'leukocytes' – these are part of the immune system that destroys and removes old or abnormal cells and cellular debris, as well as attacking infectious agents (pathogens) and foreign substances. The cancer of leukocytes is called leukaemia.
- 200,000–500,000 platelets, or 'thrombocytes' – these are responsible for blood clotting (coagulation).[i]

An average human will have 5 litres of blood which will account for about 8% of total human weight.

Incidentally, when you have a blood sample taken you are technically undergoing a biopsy. That is, it is an invasive surgical technique. When you are next asked to visit your surgery for the nurse to extract some blood you really should tell your family and friends that you are 'undergoing a biopsy' – it's almost guaranteed that you will receive much more sympathy and interest than if you say you have to give a blood sample.

It would be convenient to carry on with this explanation of what pernicious anaemia actually is without spending any more time on micro-anatomy. However, to do so would be to miss the opportunity of examining the most astonishing 'living' things in the universe – cells.

A short note on cells

Cells (of which red blood cells are just one type) are what make living things live. They were first described by a contemporary of Sir Isaac Newton, Robert Hooke, in his 1665 book *Microphagia: or Some Physiological Descriptions for Miniature Bodies Made by Magnifying Glasses*. Using his magnifying glass, he observed that plants were made up of little chambers, which he called 'cells'

---

i The very first edition of the Pernicious Anaemia Society's Newsletter was titled *The Platelet*. A haematologist suggested that this didn't mean anything and suggested it should be changed – it was changed to *Cobalamin News*.

because they looked like the small rooms, or cells, that monks used to live in. This was at the very beginning of the science of microbiology and it was a Dutchman, Antoni van Leeuwenhoek, an uneducated draper from Delft, who was responsible for ensuring that this emerging new science was placed on a firm footing. Using his remarkable early microscopes that had evolved from hand-held magnifying glasses, he began to look through a window into a new universe that was found to be teeming with life. Leeuwenhoek's microscopes worked using a single drop of water as the lens. Type 'water drop microscope' into an internet search engine and you will be directed to several websites that describe how you can make one of these truly amazing scientific instruments using clothes pegs and bits of plastic. It's hard to imagine that a drop of water, a single drop of water, could establish a whole new scientific discipline – but it did.

It was Louis Pasteur in 1864 who really set the scene for the emerging new science of biology by proving conclusively that all living matter doesn't suddenly happen spontaneously (as in maggots suddenly appearing on rotting meat), but comes from existing cells. This built on the findings of the German, Theodor Schwann, who proved that *all* living matter is made up of cells.

Cells vary in size – from nerve cells that can stretch for over a metre to our own particular favourite, the red blood cell, which is tiny. The average size of a human cell is around 20 micrometres across. Red blood cells are just 7-8 micrometres wide and 1-2 micrometres thick. They are shaped like a disc and have a concave dish on one side (see Figure 2.1). You (and I) make red blood cells in bone marrow at a rate of 2.5 million every second. Children produce red blood cells in the marrow of almost every bone in their bodies, but adults produce them only in the marrow found in the spine, ribs, pelvis and breastbone plus small parts of the upper arm and leg. Bone marrow also produces the other constituents of blood, namely the white blood cells, including platelets. Bone marrow that produces blood cells is classed as red bone marrow, and bone marrow that doesn't produce any blood cells after childhood is called yellow bone marrow. The name given to this process of producing the cells that constitute blood is 'haematopoiesis'.

Red blood cells live for about four months and then they are destroyed in the liver or spleen. They are the only cells in your body that do not contain a nucleus,[ii] at least not once they are mature; they do have a nucleus during their formative stage but this is lost as the cells age and this makes more space for haemoglobin, about which we shall learn more later.

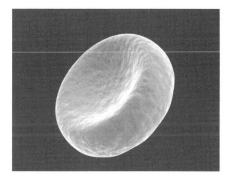

Figure 2.1 A healthy red blood cell – note the concave shape

Even though a cell, and especially a red blood cell, is incredibly small, it contains millions and millions of other objects that are so small they could be likened to ants in something the size of London's Albert Hall. These tiny objects include mitochondria, ribosomes, peroxisomes, proteins of every size and shape, endosomes and lysosomes; their precise make-up and function needn't concern us here, but they are continually bumping into each other as they enthusiastically go about their jobs of getting rid of waste, carrying out repairs, extracting energy from nutrients and dealing with intruders. Every red blood cell will have around 20,000 types of protein,[iii] with around 2,000 of

---

ii From the Latin for kernel – the centre or core of the cell – that is the 'nerve centre' of the cell.

these being made up of, at the very least, 50,000 molecules. This means that there are at least 100 million molecules of protein in each cell.

The inside of a tiny red blood cell is a very busy place. Red blood cells are important. And this is where I withdraw my toe from the water that is molecular medicine.

A short note on vitamins

In 1753 the Scottish surgeon, James Lind, published his *Treatise on the Scurvy*. Scurvy is a disease that causes bleeding spots, spongy gums, bleeding under the skin, healed wounds to re-open and teeth to fall out. It results in neuropathy (numbness), depression and suppurating wounds.[iv] Eventually it causes death. Lind had spent a number of years in the Royal Navy and it was in mariners that scurvy was mainly found. In his treatise Lind advocated preventing and treating scurvy by giving sailors citrus fruits such as lemons and limes. Incidentally, this is why Americans refer to the British as 'limeys' – because British sailors ate limes. Lind's recommendations were adopted only piecemeal by the British Navy and his work seems to have been forgotten by the late 19th century when scurvy was believed to be caused by lack of discipline, lack of exercise and poor morale. By the time of Scott's early 20th century Antarctic expeditions it was believed that 'tainted' canned food was the cause of scurvy.

What Lind had stumbled upon was that citrus foods prevented and treated a deficiency in a vitamin. At the time of his treatise nobody had even heard of vitamins and whilst other doctors began to treat various diseases such as rickets and beriberi with

---

iii Proteins are complicated compounds made up of amino acids. They play a part in almost everything a cell does. Amino acids are made up of carbon, hydrogen, oxygen and nitrogen. Any excess protein is converted into glucose and used as a source of energy.

iv The wounds emit pus.

changes to the patient's diet, nobody knew anything about vitamins themselves.

In 1884, Takaki Kanehiro, a British-trained medical doctor in the Japanese Navy, observed that beriberi, a particularly nasty disease that leads to the human body simply wasting away, was common in low-ranking crew members who ate nothing but rice. The reason for the sailors eating such a meagre diet was because these crew members were usually from poor backgrounds who, rather than spending money on healthy food, would choose to save the money to send back home. Kanehiro observed that the officers who ate a Western-style diet didn't suffer from beriberi. Dr Kanehiro either had remarkable negotiating skills or he had friends in high places, because the Japanese Navy allowed him to experiment on the crews of two battleships to test out his theory. Remarkably, the Japanese naval authorities gave the doctor access to the crew of one battleship who were fed only white rice (presumably they noticed no difference in their diet because that's what they ate anyway), while the crew of the other ship were fed meat, barley, beans, rice and fish. The white-rice-only crew had 161 crew members develop beriberi of whom 25 died, while the latter group had only 14 cases of beriberi reported and nobody died. There is no record that I can find of what the two ships were called, but LIFE and DEATH might have been appropriate names. Dr Kanehiro had proved that diet was the cause of beriberi, but mistakenly believed that sufficient amounts of protein prevented it. In fact, he had witnessed the effect of a lack of what we now know as vitamin B_1 or 'thiamine' – one of those added ingredients you find mentioned on the side of breakfast cereal boxes.

Nobody talked of vitamins yet, and it wasn't until 1912 that the magnificently named Polish doctor, Casimir Funk, building on the earlier works of Frederick Hopkins and Umetaro Suzuki, extracted water-soluble nutrients from rice bran and named it 'vitamin' – a combination of 'vital' and 'amine'. Why he chose to use the word vital is self-explanatory. The second part of the new term – amine – is the name given to a group of organic compounds that have at their base a nitrogen atom. It was believed, falsely, that nitrogen would be at the centre of all of the newly discovered vitamins.

Vitamin supplements are so widely available and used today that it is hard to imagine a world without them. Yet it was only during the early part of the 20th century that individual vitamins were identified and their true value became known.

There are two types of vitamins: those that are 'water soluble', meaning that they dissolve easily in water, and those that are 'fat soluble'; you guessed it – the fat soluble vitamins do not dissolve in water. The one that we are mostly concerned with here is vitamin B_{12}, which is water soluble. If you have somehow consumed more B_{12} than you need, it just gets passed out in your urine. You *can* overdose on water-soluble vitamins, most notably vitamin C,[v] but you would have to make a real effort to do so. Any vitamin overdose is likely to be caused by a fat-soluble vitamin. Vitamin overdose is known to doctors as 'hypervitaminosis'. There is a table in Appendix 1 which lists the vitamins, their dates of discovery and their food sources.

Vitamin B_{12}

People who are diagnosed as having pernicious anaemia will be deficient in vitamin B_{12} owing to problems in absorbing it from their food. This problem with absorbing B_{12} will be discussed later in the book, but for now we will just take a closer look at this essential vitamin.

Vitamin B_{12} is the most chemically complex of all of the vitamins. It was identified in 1926 and it is formed around a core

---

v Too much vitamin C can cause diarrhoea, nausea, flushes and, in rare cases, iron poisoning.

atom of the metal cobalt. It is produced by bacteria in the gut of ruminant animals (sheep, cows, goats) via an extremely complex chemical process. There are four companies that manufacture artificially produced B_{12} – one in France and three in China. In 2008, 35 tonnes of artificial B_{12} were produced with most of it being used to supplement animal feeds.[vi]

Artificially produced B_{12} is widely available in three forms: cyanocobalamin, hydroxocobalamin and methylcobalamin. (There is another form of B_{12} called adenosylcobalamin but this is not used to treat B_{12} deficiency because it is very unstable.)

Cyanocobalamin is available either as an injection or as a tablet. Whatever form is used, it has to be converted by the body into hydroxocobalamin. Cyanocobalamin in injection form is mainly used in North America and mainland Europe to treat patients who have B_{12} deficiency, while hydroxocobalamin is most widely used in the UK and Australia. The belief exists that hydroxocobalamin is retained in the body longer than cyanocobalamin, but the only reference I can find relating to this admits that the evidence is seriously flawed.[vii] Then the third available form of B_{12} – methylcobalamin – is what hydroxocobalamin is converted into by the body. Eventually, the body converts methylcobalamin to adenosylcobalamin. As I mentioned above, adenosylcobalamin is not widely available in artificial form, mainly due to its being very unstable – it doesn't last very long.

So, to recap, if you are injected with cyanocobalamin, your body has to convert it to hydroxocobalamin, which then has to be converted into methylcobalamin, which then has to become adenosylcobalamin. You may be wondering why people suffering from B_{12} deficiency aren't automatically treated with methylcobalamin, thereby avoiding the need for any conversion

vi This is from Wikipedia, though the external links to the original references don't work.
vii I return to this in chapter 8, see page 137.

process and thus any complications with converting the other forms of artificial B_{12}. The answer is probably to do with the cost not only of manufacturing the different types of B_{12} but also of storing them – methylcobalamin has to be kept in the dark and in a cool place. It's the form that I use to keep me alive.

So what is anaemia?

Anaemia[viii] is defined in dictionaries as a 'blood deficiency' and it is the most common blood disorder, caused by *either* a low / below average number of red blood cells[ix] in the patient's blood *or* less than the normal quantity of haemoglobin[x] in the blood.

Haemoglobin is the molecule that transports oxygen to all parts of your body – including your brain. It is made up of iron molecules – 'haem' – and other cells that form 'globin'.[xi] Red blood cells carry haemoglobin and it is the haemoglobin that is responsible for picking up and transporting oxygen. Think of there being a big red bus (the red blood cell) that is carrying passengers (the haemoglobin). The bus carrying the haemoglobin travels along a one-way system around your body called 'the vascular system', the first part of which is made up of the 'arteries'. The red buses head for the lungs, where the passengers (haemoglobin) want to go 'cruising', being on the lookout for oxygen molecules; each haemoglobin molecule can pick up not just one, but four at a time. Every so often, the haemoglobin opens the door of the bus and grabs a big balloon full of oxygen and when each passenger (haemoglobin molecule) has four balloons of oxygen the bus heads for wherever the oxygen is required – which is just about everywhere in the body. When it arrives at a place where the

viii The American spelling is without the second 'a' – anemia.
ix Often abbreviated to RBCs
x Abbreviated to Hgb or Hb
xi If you must know, it's made up of four polypeptide chains, normally two α and two non-α.

oxygen can be used, the door is opened and the oxygen balloons are thrown out. Then, molecules of carbon dioxide (CO_2) enter the bus. Yes – the carbon dioxide hangs around in the plasma before being 'picked up' by the red blood cell. The bus then heads back to the lungs via the return part of the one-way system, called the 'veins'. When the bus arrives at the lungs, the CO_2 exits the bus and is ejected from the body when the person breathes out.

This extraordinary process is taking place as you read this. That air that you have just breathed in contained oxygen. And right now that oxygen is being captured by haemoglobin that is inside your red blood cells and is being transported around your body, with some of it being deposited in the muscles responsible for you focusing your eye on this page of the book. Then that red blood cell will pick up some waste carbon dioxide and rush to your lungs, where some carbon dioxide has just been expelled in the breath you most recently exhaled. And during the time it has taken you to read this sentence, the whole process will have been repeated around 10 times.

The more energy a person uses, the more oxygen is needed and the harder the red blood cells have to work. A person performing any task that involves physical exertion will have their red blood cells working overtime. Any physical activity will require oxygen to be transported to muscles, and the more active a person is, then the more oxygen is needed, which is why we pant and breathe faster when we run – we draw in huge amounts of air, which contains oxygen. Any exertion by a person will lead to him or her automatically producing more red blood cells to ensure that there are enough of these remarkable cells around to transport the extra oxygen that is being inhaled and carry away the extra carbon dioxide that is being breathed out. Think of buses again – there are more of them around at peak commuting times, when more are needed.

It's the haemoglobin that's the important part of red blood cells when talking about anaemia. Everybody needs haemoglobin, as without it the red blood cell cannot access oxygen. If a person has fewer than the required number of red blood cells, then he or she will also be deficient in haemoglobin (because the haemoglobin makes up part of the red blood cell). But a person can have a normal quantity of red blood cells but a lower than average (or healthy) level of haemoglobin. This is because the haemoglobin molecule has, at its centre, an iron atom and if there is insufficient iron available the body cannot make sufficient quantities of hae-moglobin however many red blood cells there are. (It is interesting to note that doctors determine the amount of iron in your body by measuring your ferritin levels; ferritin is a protein that stores iron, and should not be confused with the iron itself.) So if a patient doesn't have enough iron in his/her blood (usually due to blood loss from serious wounds or menstruation), then there will not be enough haemoglobin in the red blood cell. If the number of red blood cells in a patient's blood is normal, but the amount of hae-moglobin in the red blood cells is *below* average, then the patient is diagnosed as having 'iron-deficiency anaemia' – something quite different from pernicious anaemia. Going back to the bus analogy, if a person has low iron, then the bus would be going around and around but, because there are very few or even no passengers (haemoglobin molecules) to grab the balloons full of oxygen, the oxygen cannot be captured and taken to where it is needed. There are fewer than average haemoglobin passengers on the bus because there is a shortage of iron, which is essential for the production of these passengers. It is an almost empty bus that isn't doing what it should be doing. A lack of iron leads to a lack of haemoglobin, which leads to a lack of oxygen being transported around the body – and half empty, or empty, buses.

So – a healthy person will have a normal quantity of red blood cells in their blood and those red blood cells will be carrying normal amounts of haemoglobin. If you lack one or the other, you will develop anaemia.

Haemoglobin is eventually destroyed in the liver or spleen,

but the iron part of the molecule is removed and stored. Most of the 'leftovers' from the destruction of red cells in your liver are re-cycled for further use.[xii]

Iron-deficient anaemia may be attributable to diet and can usually be corrected by taking iron tablets – sometimes prescribed by doctors. There are many other causes of anaemia, but all apart from pernicious anaemia are beyond the scope of this book, and the science involved is, quite frankly, beyond me.

The role of vitamin B$_{12}$

So where does vitamin B$_{12}$ come into all of this? Well, vitamin B$_{12}$ is vital for the formation of normal red blood cells. When the red blood cell is being made, vitamin B$_{12}$ is an essential component in the construction process. Without vitamin B$_{12}$ two things happen when the red blood cell is being formed. Firstly, without vitamin B$_{12}$, red blood cells become enlarged and change shape in that they lose the concave little dish that is so important in allowing the cell to transport oxygen. Secondly, it will be a faulty cell that is produced and it won't last very long. Think of the bus analogy – if a crucial part is missing during the production of the bus, then the bus will be unreliable and will not go very far before breaking down. That's why vitamin B$_{12}$ is so important. Without it the essential red blood cells will be faulty and unable to do what they should – carry oxygen to wherever it is needed and dispose of carbon dioxide – the fundamental work of blood. Vitamin B$_{12}$ is a very important vitamin.

An average human being has an enormous number of red blood cells – they account for around a quarter of all cells in your

xii The Pernicious Anaemia Society has published a paper on this written by one of our members, Mr Kevin Byrne – *The Enterohepatic Circulation of B12*. It is available in two formats – one in plain English and one aimed at medical professionals. This 'mopping up' of the left-overs of destroyed red blood cells will become an important discussion topic later on.

body[1] – and you make an awful lot of them – around 2.4 million every second;[3] that's quite a production line that not even the most advanced motor manufacturing plant could equal if we remember the red bus analogy. As we know, red blood cells are made in bone marrow and take around seven days to be produced. They then go about doing what they are designed to do, which is carry oxygen to wherever it is needed, and, after around 100 to 120 days, they are recycled. And this all goes on without us having to trouble ourselves to do anything special – it all happens automatically. You'll never hear someone say, 'Excuse me, I have to go and make some red blood cells,' and if you ever do, you'll need seriously to review the subject matter of the conversation you were having. From the day you are born you automatically produce these little marvels without having ever to think about it.

So, to recap, people who lack vitamin B_{12} cannot produce healthy red blood cells. And, consequently, their red blood cells cannot do what they are supposed to do, which is to carry oxygen around the body to wherever it is needed.

Eating foods that contain B_{12} is, therefore, essential to ensure that we make healthy red blood cells. In the next chapter we will investigate what foods contain B_{12} and in what quantities.

References

1   Laura Dean. *Blood Groups and Red Cell Antigens* National Center for Biotechnology Information (NCBI), National Library of Medicine, National Institutes of Health, Bethesda, MD 20892-6510, 2005.
2   Pierigè F, Serafini S, Rossi L, Magnani M (January 2008). Cell-based drug delivery. *Advanced Drug Delivery Reviews* **60**(2): 286–95. doi:10.1016/j.addr.2007.08.029. PMID 17997501.
3   Erich Sackmann. Biological Membranes Architecture and Function. In: *Handbook of Biological Physics* (Edited by Lipowsky R and Sackmann E) vol. 1, London: Elsevier, 1995.

Chapter 3

Sources of vitamin B$_{12}$

In November 2011, I asked 10 people, chosen at random in a supermarket car park, if they believed that a balanced diet was the best kind of diet. All 10 of those questioned stated quite categorically that a balanced diet was indeed the best. The UK government's campaign to promote the benefits of a healthy balanced diet has obviously worked. However, when asked to explain what a healthy diet actually meant, all 10 interviewees stated that a balanced diet revolved around eating five portions of fruit and vegetables every day. Not one mentioned the need for meat or dairy products in their diet, which are the main sources of vitamin B$_{12}$. (I would have asked more but I was told by the security guard that I would need written permission from the manager to conduct any sort of interviews on the supermarket's premises.) Whilst five portions of fruit and vegetables may be *part* of a balanced diet, so are fish, meat and dairy products if you are to avoid being deficient in B$_{12}$. And we know from the previous chapter just how important B$_{12}$ is. Vitamin B$_{12}$ is such an important factor in ensuring good health that it is essential every person gets a sufficient supply of the vitamin to enable the production of healthy red blood cells. So how do we ensure that we get enough B$_{12}$?

Vitamin B$_{12}$ is found in all animal products – meat, fish and dairy produce, including cheese, butter and milk. There are foods, supposedly healthy foods, which contain no B_{12} whatsoever – fruit and vegetables being the most notable. No matter how many apples you eat, no matter how many sticks of celery you consume, and no matter how many carrots you can digest, no essential vitamin B_{12} can be extracted from them.

The UK's Food Standards Agency is the government agency responsible for ensuring that the food we eat in the UK is of a sufficiently high standard to keep people well. The agency issues regulations and guidelines for the manufacture and distribution of all the different foods that we eat and it also maintains the UK Nutrient Databank that lists 3,423 different foodstuffs and gives all the nutritional data on those foods that you could possibly want. It proudly boasts that 'the data are divided across 16 worksheets and include nutrient data for macronutrients, vitamins, vitamin fractions, minerals, fatty acid fractions, phytosterols,[i] and organic acids, as well as providing recalculated values for a selection of foods in the format required for nutrition labelling'. These data sets are a fascinating source of information and I once spent a whole afternoon just scanning them to find out what different foods contain. The amount of information about supposedly simple foods is staggering. The datasets are more correctly called the *McCance and Widdowson's The Composition of Foods (CoF) book series*. You have to take your hat off to McCance and Widdowson for beginning the work that still bears their names – the very first study was begun in the 1930s, not long after vitamins were discovered. There are 16 sets of data overall but the one that interests us will be the datasheet on the vitamin content of ordinary foods. Here, under the column labelled 'U', we can find which foods can provide the consumer with decent amounts of the vitamin that we are concerned with – B_{12}.

---

i Phystosterols are found in plants and vegetable oils and have been proven to lower cholesterol.

Before I provide you with a sample of the vitamin B_{12} content of these different foodstuffs, we need to examine the quantities involved. A team of highly dedicated scientists sampled 100 grams of edible portions of each food. A gram is a small amount – a small paperclip is about one gram – so the total weight of the edible portion would weigh the same as 100 paperclips. I've just conducted a short survey of household objects to find an everyday item that weighs around 100 grams. My *Bridget Jones's Diary* CD in its hard plastic case weighs almost exactly 100 grams, while the DVD of Michael Jackson's *This Is It* falls just short of 100 grams. My Blackberry Curve mobile phone weighs 105 grams. An average packet of butter is 250 grams, so a 'knob of butter' as used by television chefs will probably amount to 100 grams – TV chefs' idea of a knob of butter is different from the average cook's portion.

The amount of B_{12} in each of the 100 gram food portions is given in micrograms, which is often written as 'μg' or 'mcg' and is one millionth of a gram.[ii]

How much B_{12} should we get every day?

Astonishingly, there is no agreement as to how much B_{12} an average adult should consume on a daily basis. The United Kingdom's *NHS Choices* website states that the recommended daily intake of B_{12} is 1.5 micrograms per day while the United States' Office of Dietary Supplements recommends a daily intake of 2.4 micrograms.[1] Vitamin supplements and cereal packets also have varying figures. Health Canada states that the minimum intake for an adult should be 2.4 micrograms per day, with that increasing to a very precise 2.6 micrograms per day for a

---

ii The US-based Joint Commission on Accreditation of Healthcare Organizations recommends using mcg instead of the μ symbol on patients' notes and records because of the risk of the μ being mistaken for an 'm' which could lead to a 1000-fold overdose of whatever medicine is being prescribed.

pregnant woman – the difference between an average human's intake of B_{12} and a pregnant woman being an almost immeasurable 0.2 of a millionth of a gram. An article in the *American Journal of Clinical Nutrition* from 2006 found that, 'A daily vitamin B-12 intake of 6 μg appeared to be sufficient to correct all the vitamin B-12–related variables measured in the postmenopausal Danish women'[2] – in effect, recommending 6 micrograms every day to ensure that there are no B_{12} deficiency problems in women who have undergone the menopause. Some of the participants in the study were given 14 micrograms per day – but the researchers found that this made no difference to the level of B_{12} in the blood from those who were given 6 micrograms daily.

The American Institute of Medicine publishes the *Dietary Reference Intakes for Thiamin,*[iii] *Riboflavin, Niacin, Vitamin B_6, Folate, Vitamin B_{12}, Pantothenic Acid, Biotin, and Choline,*[3] and the 1998 edition states:

'The median intake of vitamin B_{12} from food in the United States was estimated to be approximately 5 μg/day for men and 3.5 μg/day for women. The ninety-fifth percentile of vitamin B_{12} intake from both food and supplements was approximately 27 μg/day. In one Canadian province, the mean dietary intake was estimated to be approximately 7 μg/day for men and 4 μg/day for women. There is not sufficient scientific evidence to set a tolerable upper intake level (UL) for vitamin B_{12} at this time.'

Let's settle on an average human needing around 2 micrograms of B_{12} every day, and if anyone takes more than that they will have to face the consequences of doing so – which are none.

So what foods are the best sources of B_{12}? Well, Messrs McCance and Widdowson start their mammoth task of identifying and calculating the amount of vitamins in everyday food by analysing

iii The UK places an 'e' at the end – 'thiamine' – otherwise known as vitamin B_1.

beer – perhaps they needed some liquid refreshment to ease them into their endeavours. The data sheet for vitamins has four indicators – the figure 0 denotes there is absolutely no B_{12} present in that particular food; T stands for 'trace', meaning that there is some B_{12} in the foodstuff but the figure is so small that it cannot be reliably weighed; figures in brackets are estimates of the amount of B_{12} in the food, and then finally there's the more reliable and trustworthy numerical value. The good news is that Guinness is indeed good for you – but only in the sense that it contains a trace of B_{12}. And that means that no matter how much of it you drink, you will not get your recommended daily intake before your liver will give up on you. Egg nog, though, has 0.9 micrograms of B_{12}.

The detail which the tables give about the samples of food analysed are really intriguing. Take, for example, the investigation of what vitamins are contained in black tea. The authors didn't just sample black tea – they differentiated between *weak* black tea and *strong* black tea.

Tea, black, infusion, weak	10 grams leaves per litre water, strained after 5 minutes; 10 samples
Tea, black, infusion, strong	10 grams leaves per 500 millilitres water, strained after 5 minutes; 10 samples

Whether you like your tea strong or weak, the B_{12} content is the same – 0.00 micrograms. The same is true for coffee, and the biscuits that you may take with your beverage of choice. Nor is there any to be found in bread (with the exception of wholemeal where a trace can be found, though when toasted it surprisingly yields 0.7 micrograms). Poppadums, jam tarts, 'Asian pastries' and ciabatta do not have any B_{12}. Breakfast cereals nearly all contain added B_{12} along with other vitamins and minerals, the exceptions being wheat biscuits and puffed wheat. Breakfast cereals tell you on the box what the vitamin content is because the cereals are *fortified* – which is to say that they have vitamins added to them during their manufacture. Why breakfast cereals have been singled out to have vitamins added to them, with other foodstuffs being ignored, is a question I have been unable to find an answer to. For two weeks in the summer of 2011 while researching this book I found that I couldn't pass a display of breakfast cereals without scanning their content and finding out which had been fortified. Family members and friends thought I was sad – I found it fascinating.

If you were to buy some beef steak you wouldn't be able to read how much B_{12} it contains simply because none has been *added* – it is naturally part of the meat. Breakfast cereals, or most of them, have had vitamins, including B_{12}, added to them.

To find out how much 'naturally occurring' B_{12} is in different food-stuffs you can rely on McCance and Widowson's remarkable tables. According to these, 100 grams of a tuna mayonnaise sandwich on white bread gets you 1.4 micrograms because it contains an animal product – both tuna and the mayonnaise, which is made from egg yolks. Remember, that's based on the standard 100 grams of the sandwich. A duck egg (raw) delivers 5.4 micrograms, but please don't eat raw duck eggs. Surprisingly, given their source, lard, butter and beef dripping only have a trace of B_{12}.

Sea-foods, especially shellfish, are a good source of B_{12}. A hundred grams of boiled prawns are estimated to contain 8 micrograms; sardines canned in tomato sauce provide a whopping 14 micrograms. Similarly, boiled mussels have 22 micrograms, while boiled cockles provide a healthy 47 micrograms of B_{12}.

Meat extract (such as Bovril) has 7 micrograms of B_{12} while yeast extract – such as Marmite – has just 1 microgram of B_{12}, but is rich in other B vitamins including folate.[iv] Just to muddy the waters, this differs from what is stated on the jar of Marmite itself. Meat

---

iv Otherwise known as folic acid or vitamin B_9 – which is routinely given to pregnant mothers to prevent neural tube defects in the foetus.

itself doesn't score extremely highly: it's a good source of B_{12}. 100 grams of homemade hamburger contain only 2.4 micrograms, while chicken breast marinated in garlic contains only a trace of the vitamin. Fried sirloin steak contains 2 micrograms and, rather surprisingly, rump steak has more – 3 micrograms. Don't forget these are figures for 100 grams of the meat. Ten Chinese takeaways were visited in the name of nutritional science and the crispy duck was analysed – it contained 2–8 micrograms of B_{12}.

One foodstuff that promises to contain high amounts of B_{12} is black pudding, which is made from pigs' blood. It yields a disappointing 2 micrograms – mainly because the B_{12} is used in the manufacture of red blood cells and so most will have already been used up by the animal, although some would have still been present in the animal's blood.

It's offal that is the big hitter for B_{12} content. Figures from shellfish are dwarfed in comparison to offal – often the cheapest meat at the butcher's counter. A hundred grams of haggis contains 2 micrograms of B_{12}, stewed liver and onions contains 29.7 micrograms – more than 10 times your recommended daily intake. Fried lamb's kidney has 54 micrograms; fried lamb's liver has 83 micrograms, whilst stewed ox liver contains 110 micrograms of B_{12}.

You don't have to eat offal to get your full 2.5 micrograms of B_{12} either. One hundred grams of cheddar cheese, which is quite a hefty chunk, has the full recommended daily intake, as does a cheese omelette, whilst a glass of semi-skimmed milk contains just short of 1 microgram, and milk chocolate has a rounded 1 microgram. A hundred grams of a McDonald's cheeseburger contains 2 micrograms – nearly a day's worth of B_{12}. Cauliflower cheese contains 0.5 micrograms. Carrot halva yields 0.9 micrograms, raw sheep's milk 0.6 micrograms (again I am not recommending that you try raw sheep's milk), vanilla ice cream 0.5, whilst 100 grams of pressed tongue gets you 5 micrograms of B_{12} – double your daily requirement.

You don't have to eat foodstuffs that contain B_{12} every day as you store around 2,500 micrograms, mostly in blood in your liver.[v] This is why the symptoms of B_{12} deficiency are insidious – they creep up on the patient very slowly unlike many other diseases where the symptoms manifest themselves quickly. Because of the insidious way in which the symptoms appear they are often attributed, by the patient and the physician, to the natural ageing process, or the consequence of a hectic modern lifestyle. They are often ignored for many years as the patient just learns to live with them. This is why many people who have the symptoms of B_{12} deficiency can and do go on to develop irreversible nerve damage. And all of this is because it takes a long time to completely deplete the patient's stores of B_{12} held in his or her body.

With the vitamin being so ubiquitous in modern diets, it's hard to explain why there is so much vitamin B_{12} deficiency, yet there are professionals (for example, Smith and Refsum, see pages 41 to 42) who believe that B_{12} deficiency is much more common than has been previously assumed and the symptoms are often associated with other illnesses, leading to misdiagnosis by medical professionals and consequent misery for the patient.

Now you'd think that just by eating any food that contains B_{12} a normal healthy person would be able to avoid B_{12} deficiency. To a certain extent that is true, but there's something else that needs to be taken into account. Surprisingly, some foodstuffs containing B_{12} are more 'biologically available' than others. This means that some foods that contain the same amount of B_{12} as others, are able to give up their B_{12} more easily to the complex biological process that sees the B_{12} absorbed into the blood stream.

A large study carried out on 5,937 Norwegian people found that:

---

v It is commonly believed that B_{12} is stored in the liver; however, there are doctors who refute this. As this is an argument that is only just beginning, I don't want to get involved in it.

'Plasma vitamin B-12 was associated with intakes of increasing amounts of vitamin B-12 from dairy products or fish… but not with intakes of vitamin B-12 from meat or eggs. For the same content of vitamin B-12, intake from dairy products led to the greatest increase in plasma vitamin B-12. Total intake of vitamin B-12, particularly from milk and fish, decreased the risk of vitamin B-12 concentrations <200 pmol/L and impaired vitamin B-12 function (vitamin B-12 <200 pmol/L and methylmalonic acid .0.27 lmol/L) in the total group and in 71–74-y-old subjects'.[4]

In short, fish and dairy products are better at preventing B_{12} deficiency than meat and eggs. The report concludes:

'In conclusion, we suggest that, even in a well-nourished population, dietary intake is an important contributor to plasma vitamin B-12. It appears that vitamin B-12 in meat is less bioavailable than is that in milk and fish, which may have implications for recommendations about how to maintain a good vitamin B-12 status. On the basis of our observations and of previously published findings ... it seems that daily dietary vitamin B-12 intake between 6 and 10 µg ensures the maximal plasma vitamin B-12 concentration in persons with adequate vitamin B-12 absorption. This amount is considerably larger than the current recommended daily intake. We suggest that the guidelines for improving vitamin B-12 status should focus on the intake of dairy products, particularly milk, because vitamin B-12 appears to be more bioavailable from these sources'.[4]

This is a remarkable conclusion. Firstly, it states that the recommended daily dietary intake of B_{12} be raised from the current level of around 2 micrograms per day to between three and five times that number and that dairy products are nutritionally important – something that flies in the face of some contemporary advice.

One group of people who are obviously in danger of being

deficient in B_{12} are vegetarians, especially vegans.[vi] What might be glaringly obvious from what we know about the sources of B_{12} – that people who don't eat any animal products will consequently be deficient in vitamin B_{12} – is, however, not necessarily true. Strict vegans do not wash vegetables and so will absorb some vitamin B_{12} from the soil attached to root vegetables. Thomas E Billings, who runs the website *Beyond Vegetarianism*,[5] states, in his article, 'Is a strict, 100% vegan diet optimal (for everyone)?':

'A vegan diet needs a reliable source of vitamin B_{12}. Plant foods can contain some vitamin B_{12}, which is absorbed from soil and water (Mozafar 1994).[6] However, the amount varies with the B-12 content of the soil (some soil has no B_{12}), so plant foods alone are not a reliable source (Billings 1999).[7] A group of vegan nutritionists recommends that vegans take B_{12} supplements or consume (processed) foods fortified with B_{12} (Walsh 2001).[8] Some advocates suggest regular blood testing and using supplements only if indicated, an approach that appears over-cautious given the low cost and safety record of B_{12} supplementation.'

Small amounts of B_{12} might occur in plants under some circumstances if they have been grown in soil rich in manure, but this is not a common finding and vegans should in no way rely on getting B_{12} from plants, even from vegetables grown organically.

The last sentence of Billings's short explanation is the most pertinent to this book's following chapters and I cannot emphasise enough how important it is; he doesn't go along with the 'vegan nutritionists' who advocate regular blood tests for vegans as this is an 'over-cautious approach' because of the 'low cost and safety record of B_{12} supplementation'. In other words, don't bother with

---

vi By vegetarians I mean those that eat neither fish nor meat but may consume eggs or dairy products or both. Some vegetarians consume fish while others eat meat only very rarely.

blood tests; just take supplements of B_{12} as they will not do you any harm. This is a subject that will keep raising its head as we continue through this investigation of the way vitamin B_{12} deficiency in general, and pernicious anaemia in particular, are diagnosed and treated. What's clear is that vegans and vegetarians need to take B_{12} supplements if they are to avoid suffering from B_{12} deficiency. They're cheap and there is no risk of suffering any side effects.

The British Geological Survey (BGS) has produced a map that identifies areas of England and Wales where there is very little or no cobalt in the soil (see Figure 3.1). It also indicates where there are healthy levels. Why would anyone want to investigate

Figure 3.1 Map showing the levels of cobalt in soil in England and Wales courtesy of the British Geological Survey (BGS) and the National Soil Inventory (NSI)

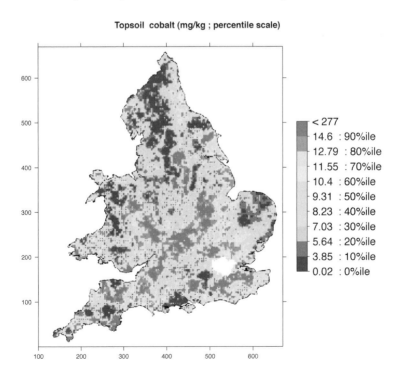

Topsoil cobalt (mg/kg ; percentile scale)

< 277
14.6 : 90%ile
12.79 : 80%ile
11.55 : 70%ile
10.4 : 60%ile
9.31 : 50%ile
8.23 : 40%ile
7.03 : 30%ile
5.64 : 20%ile
3.85 : 10%ile
0.02 : 0%ile

the concentration levels of cobalt in soil in different geographical areas? This was the question that I put to Dr Neil Breward of the BGS, who told me:

> 'BGS has carried out geochemical surveys for a wide range of elements of economic, environmental and geoscientific interest in stream sediments, stream waters and soils. These include several elements of major importance in agriculture/animal health, including cobalt, molybdenum and copper. Geochemical maps of the concentration of such elements enable areas of potential excess or deficiency to be identified for further detailed examination.'

It's good to know that someone is keeping an eye on the amount of cobalt in soil, but I couldn't help wondering if there is a relationship between these and B_{12} deficiency in animals. I asked Neil if B_{12} deficiency in animals could be related to low cobalt levels in soil and he replied:

> 'Almost certainly, but it is a complex matter involving not just low total levels of cobalt, but several other soil factors and translocation issues too. Certainly, there will be a greater risk of animal B_{12} deficiency in areas where grazing is co-deficient due to very low soil cobalt content, but in the UK at least, soil cobalt levels are rarely below the tentative threshold value required for serious deficiency. This is more of a well-defined problem in other parts of the world. This link requires serious professional scientific investigation.'

Cobalt makes up the core of the molecule cobalamin, otherwise known as vitamin B_{12} – remember it's the only vitamin that has a metal as its core. Ruminants (cows, sheep and goats) produce B_{12} in the rumen (part of the stomach), where bacteria use cobalt to produce the vitamin.

It is well established that ruminants, especially sheep, can become B_{12} deficient in areas where the cobalt level in soil is low – grazing animals need to ingest cobalt to allow the bacteria in their stomach to do their job and produce the B_{12} which is formed around the cobalt atom. This is an important point – animals that do not eat other animals produce vitamin B_{12} in their stomachs using bacteria. Cobalt-deficient soil is a serious problem in parts of Australia and 'cobalt licks' are provided in fields where they graze. The same is true in a few parts of the UK. Sheep, in particular, suffer from 'pine' – a disease caused by lack of cobalt and consequent lack of B_{12}. The symptoms of pine are that the sheep will just stare at the ground and not do very much – something that people who have experienced B_{12} deficiency can empathise with.

Another aspect of B_{12} in soil is that large amounts of fishmeal are used by farmers as fertiliser. Fishmeal is made up of the ground-up flesh, bones and offal of fish and other marine life. To quote Miles & Chapman of the University of Florida, it contains, among other things, large amounts of B_{12}:

'Fishmeal is considered to be a moderately rich source of vitamins of the B-complex especially cobalamin (B_{12}), niacin, choline, pantothenic acid, and riboflavin'.[9]

Fishmeal is also regularly fed to pigs.

Judging by the amount of B_{12} in processed foods, including the hugely popular breakfast cereals consumed in vast amounts every day in the Western and developing worlds, you would have to try hard to be deficient in the vitamin. Yet some authorities think that vitamin B_{12} deficiency is more widespread than is commonly believed. I asked Professor David Smith, Emeritus Professor of Pharmacology at the University of Oxford, if he was aware of any issues with B_{12} in the general population. This is what he had to say:

'Low vitamin B_{12} status is more common than generally recognised, both by the population and by GPs, at any stage of life and

not only in the elderly. The traditional diagnostic criteria that only require anaemia or changes to the blood cells are not sufficient since severe and irreversible harm can occur, especially to the nervous system, without detectable changes in the blood cells. Unfortunately, it is not generally recognised in the UK that low-normal levels of B_{12} might cause harm.'

And so, it seems, there are problems with recognising the symptoms of B_{12} deficiency – which is what we will look at next. Oh, and by the way, the *Bridget Jones* soundtrack isn't mine; it's my wife's.

Diminishing nutrients[10]

In 1991 McCance and Widdowson were asked to compare the current results of the chemical composition of food with those that they produced in the 1940s. The result of the comparison showed that the nutritional content of food had severely diminished in just 50 years. Whilst there had been some changes in the way in which the foods were analysed, the authors assured the Medical Research Council that had commissioned the work that the old methods of analysis were 'no less accurate than the modern automated ones, but they took a much longer time'. They examined 28 raw vegetables, 44 cooked vegetables, 17 fruits and 10 types of meat, poultry and game. What they found was quite staggering. This is a list of the greatest mineral losses measured in milligrams for every 100 grams between the 1940s samples and those taken in the early 1990s:

FOOD	LOSS
Carrots	75% less magnesium, 48% less calcium, 46% less iron and 75% less copper
Broccoli (boiled)	75% less calcium
Spring onion	74% less calcium
Spinach (boiled)	60% less iron and 96% less copper
Swede	71% less iron
Watercress	93% less copper
Potatoes	30% less magnesium, 35% less calcium, 45% less iron, 47% less copper
All meats	41% less calcium and 54% less iron
Apples and oranges	67% less iron
All fruits	27% less zinc

The authors of the report pointed out that you would have to eat 10 tomatoes in 1991 to get the same copper as one tomato would have given you in 1940 or three oranges to get the iron you would have got in one orange 50 years previously.

We have already seen that iron plays an important part in the manufacture of healthy red blood cells. Spinach is an excellent source of iron, and folic acid, another important player in producing red blood cells. In 1948 there were 158 milligrams of iron in 100 grams of spinach, but this had fallen to 2.2 milligrams by the early 1990s. I cannot find the corresponding figures for folic acid, but Popeye would have to eat some 200 cans of spinach today to get the same strengthening effects of iron that he would have got from just one can 60 years ago.

References

1   Office of Dietary Supplements – The National Institutes of Health: http://ods.od.nih.gov/factsheets/VitaminB12/

2   Bor MV, Lydeking-Olsen E, Møller J, Nexø E. A daily intake of approximately 6µg vitamin B-12 appears to saturate all the vitamin B-12-related variables in Danish postmenopausal women. *American Journal of Clinical Nutrition* 2006;. 83(1): 52-58.

3   American Institute of Medicine. *Dietary reference intakes for thiamine, riboflavin, niacin, vitamin B6, folate, vitamin B12, pantothenic acid, biotin and choline.* US: National Academies Press; Pap/Cdr edition (Jun 2003).

4   Vogiatzoglou AV, Smith AD, Nurk E, et al. Dietary sources of vitamin B-12 and their association with plasma vitamin B-12 concentrations in the general population: the Hordaland Homocysteine Study1–3. *American Journal of Clinical Nutrition* 2009; 89: 1078–1087.

5   Billings TE. Is a strict 100% vegan diet optimal (for everyone)? *Beyond Vegetarianism* www.beyondveg.com [full URL? Year?]

6   Mozafar A. Enrichment of some B-vitamins in plants with application of organic fertilizers. *Plant and Soil* 1994: 167; 305-311.

7   Billings TE. Vitamin B-12: Rhetoric and reality, part 4 of: Comparative anatomy and physiology brought pp to date. *Beyond Vegetarianism* 1999 www.beyondveg.com/billings-t/comp-anat/comp-anat-7d.shtml

8   Walsh S. What every vegan should know about vitamin B12. *Beyond Vegetarianism* [year?]www.beyondveg.com/walsh-s/vitamin-b12/vegans-1.shtml

9   Miles RD, Chapman FA. The benefits of fish meal in aquaculture diets. July 2006 www.thefishsite.com/articles/200/the-benefits-of-fish-meal-in-aquaculture-diets

10 Vitamin supplements – and why we need them. *What Doctors don't Tell You* 2002: 13 (9) www.wddty.co.uk

Chapter 4

The symptoms of B$_{12}$ deficiency

People who have been diagnosed with pernicious anaemia will by definition be deficient in vitamin B$_{12}$. The reason for their deficiency is a biological malfunction that we will explore in chapter 6. It is the symptoms of this deficiency that we shall examine now.

In July 2010, the Pernicious Anaemia Society produced a questionnaire that all existing members were invited to complete online. Once the member had completed the questionnaire it couldn't be completed by the same person again. All new members were asked to complete it when they first visited the website. Members who were not online members – otherwise known as 'paper members' – were all sent a hard copy to complete and their results were fed into the online version. Nearly 1,000 members have now completed the questionnaire, which was designed by a GP who is a sufferer and a member of the society – Dr Fiona Porter-Smith. Dr Porter-Smith is currently busy analysing this unique dataset and the results will be published soon. As we continue our journey investigating the problems with, and consequences of, the symptoms, diagnosis and treatment of pernicious anaemia and B$_{12}$ deficiency, I will be referring, where appropriate, to the preliminary findings of the survey.

There are four main problems with the symptoms of B$_{12}$ deficiency, which I will discuss in this chapter: they develop slowly over time, sometimes over many years; they are described in textbooks and other conventional reference sources only in vague,

*Figure 4.1 PA Society Questionnaire – Chart showing the **general symptoms** experienced by the survey respondents (courtesy of the Pernicious Anaemia Society)*

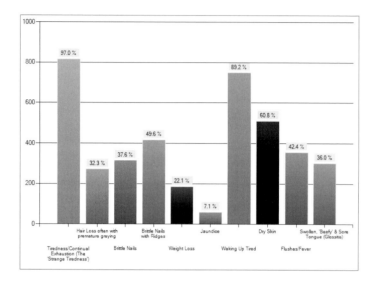

non-specific terms; some important, quite specific symptoms have until now not been recognised; and – most frustratingly of all – the symptoms usually do not go away once treatment has started, though logic would dictate that they should. I shall look at each of these problem areas in turn.

Slow development of symptoms

The symptoms of pernicious anaemia and vitamin B_{12} deficiency are insidious in that they don't appear suddenly but creep up on the patient over a long period of time – often over many years. Because they appear only gradually, the patient will often learn to live with them and make small adjustments to his or her life to accommodate and deal with them. For example, he or she will often not associate any tiredness that they are experiencing with an illness, but will believe that it is related to age or lifestyle, so he or she will not mention this slowly increasing fatigue when visiting their doctor. The patient will go to bed a little earlier, cut back on strenuous pastimes and generally make allowances for being tired. Because the tiredness doesn't suddenly manifest itself it is not associated with any disease. Likewise, any shortage of breath, memory loss, or problems with concentrating can all be attributed to advancing years – especially as these symptoms will not have appeared suddenly, but will have gradually developed over a number of years. Even if the patient does mention the fact that he or she is tired all the time to his/her doctor, the doctor may well just sympathise and tell the patient that he or she is also tired due to the demands of modern medical practice.

I remember when I first started to experience a dull tiredness and fatigue that wouldn't go away. I started to wake up tired and couldn't shrug it off. As I stated earlier, I had a hectic lifestyle and, because the tiredness didn't suddenly appear, but began to make everyday living just that tiny bit more difficult over many months, I attributed it to my reaching 40 and I remember thinking that it was all downhill from here and all that I had to look forward to was developing liver spots. I didn't mention it to my doctor even when I was being investigated for nerve damage and undergoing tests to establish why my legs were numb and my balance was deteriorating. By the time the patient considers this continual tiredness to be more than attributable to natural ageing or lifestyle, he or she is usually severely deficient in an essential vitamin and really quite ill.

How symptoms are described

The second major problem is that the symptoms that are listed in medical textbooks are generally vague and not in any way associated specifically with pernicious anaemia or B_{12} deficiency – they are often associated with a myriad of other diseases and conditions and the way they are described hasn't changed for nearly 100 years. Over the past three years, online discussions, user panels and focus groups with members of the Pernicious Anaemia Society have identified much more accurate and specific descriptions of the symptoms. Adopting these newly developed descriptions that could replace the archaic and vague symptoms currently used by medical professionals would probably lead to a quicker and more accurate diagnosis of B_{12} deficiency. What follows is a brief explanation of each established symptom together with more specific terminology to describe that symptom more accurately or more specifically.

Tiredness/lethargy

'Tiredness' only goes a little way to describing how a patient with B_{12} deficiency feels. Ordinary tiredness can be cured by sleep or perhaps small adjustments to everyday activities. For a great many patients with pernicious anaemia, sleep does not relieve the constant exhaustion. Sleep patterns vary from patient to patient, but even after 12 hours' sleep I still feel tired. Often members of the Society will tell me that they could just spend the rest of their lives in bed, and this feeling of continual weariness leads to lethargy, and the patient having no enthusiasm for life. Rachael is aged 27 and is a primary school teacher. She was diagnosed two years ago after suffering the continual tiredness for three years: 'I come home from school and just go straight upstairs to my bed where I remain for at least 12 hours,' she told me on the telephone. 'My family and friends don't understand and I am really struggling with my job.'

The online focus group came up with a much more accurate phrase to describe the tiredness experienced by sufferers – we now call it 'the strange tiredness'[i] because it is not like normal

---

i This was identified by a young teenage member of the online focus group who suggested it as a description of the inadequate 'tiredness' – it was immediately adopted by those taking part.

tiredness. It is more 'intense' and it becomes your unwelcome friend if you experience it. What makes it even more complicated is that this symptom affects people to varying degrees. Some are unable to work, play a full part in family life, hold onto relationships or have any social life. Others will manage to do all of the above but always performing at less than full capacity and always under a cloud of fatigue.

And now is the time to reveal that for a great many sufferers, the strange tiredness does not go away – even after treatment has begun. For others, the strange tiredness does recede and sometimes disappears completely. Why the B_{12} replacement therapy relieves this debilitating symptom in some and not others has not been explained by doctors, although many know that this is the case. The worst case of this tiredness affecting people's lives involves young people. It is heart-breaking to hear of individuals in their early 20s having relationship problems because they are too tired to have a normal social life, being unable to cope with the demands of college education, dropping out, and being labelled 'lazy' by their teachers, family and friends. This leads to a feeling of isolation and, yes, depression, although this is not due to anything other than the strange tiredness that won't go away even after treatment.

No research has as yet been done to find out why a person who is being treated for B_{12} deficiency may still experience this continual tiredness even after he or she has had their B_{12} deficiency corrected by injections. Instead, clinicians point to the now healthy level of B_{12} in a patient's blood and conclude that the patient is either imagining the symptoms or is depressed. I have discussed the reason why a great many of the members of the Pernicious Anaemia Society are still symptomatic after treatment has been started with medical professionals and their response is nearly always that the patient must be imagining the tiredness, although a few have hinted that they may be suffering from another, yet unidentified disease that has developed as a consequence of the patient having been B_{12} deficient for a long time. One haematologist suggested that it is all to do with scarring on the patient's brain due to the deficiency in the past. What is certain is that the patients who are still continually tired, to one extent or another, are not imagining it – there are simply far too many members of the Society who are still symptomatic even after treatment to correct their B_{12} deficiency has begun.

Another way in which this strange tiredness can be described is that the patient often complains of 'waking up tired', even after many hours' sleeping.

Shortage of breath

This is a common textbook symptom and relates to the patient having to breathe faster in order to try to provide enough oxygen for the blood to transport to where it is needed. Because the red blood cells are faulty and unable to do this, the instinctive reaction of the body is to provide more oxygen via the lungs by breathing faster. Actually, I know of nobody with pernicious anaemia who is continually panting in an effort to absorb more oxygen. And because a patient doesn't puff and pant when consulting his/her doctor, the doctor will assume that this important indicator of B_{12} deficiency is not evident. Actually, a patient with suspected pernicious anaemia will have breathing problems, but they will not involve panting – it will be displayed as sighing, otherwise identified by the online focus group as 'the sighs'. If you are reading this and you have B_{12} deficiency, you will probably be nodding your head while you are reading this. 'The sighs' is a much more accurate description of the breathing problems than the usually attributed 'shortage of breath'. This is because, while sufferers will instinctively try to compensate for the lack of oxygen being transported around their bodies by the malformed red blood cells by taking in more oxygen, they do so by increasing the *volume* of air being drawn in rather than by fast shallow breaths – they take continual deep breaths or sighs. This is the reason why many members of the Pernicious Anaemia Society are also to be seen continually yawning – especially during the afternoons – and yes, it is contagious, especially among other sufferers. Again, doctors are unable to explain why, if the patient's blood contains healthy amounts of B_{12} and, consequently, a normal number of red blood cells, he or she is instinctively trying to provide more oxygen to the lungs. Just because doctors don't know why this is so doesn't mean that it doesn't happen: just observe the breathing of onetime B_{12} deficient people – they continually sigh even though the amount of B_{12}, red blood cells and haemoglobin are healthy, though more on some days than others.

Confusion & memory problems

This is another classic textbook set of symptoms and is again often associated with advancing years. These mental issues are known to sufferers as 'the fogs'. It is no coincidence that the documentary that the Society produced in 2011 was called *Living With The Fog*. Nothing comes closer to describing how it feels trying to concentrate with B_{12} deficiency than 'living in the fog'. It describes what everyday living with pernicious anaemia is like – not only before diagnosis and treatment but also, unfortunately, for a great many sufferers, after treatment has been started.

There are other associated symptoms that are due to problems with the brain not functioning properly (see Figure 4.2). 'Nominal aphasia' is a common consequence of B_{12} deficiency and occurs even after treatment has begun – it's forgetting the names of common everyday objects or the names of family members, work colleagues or even actors or newsreaders on television or radio. I remember that I was out walking one day before I was diagnosed and staring at some sheep in a field – we have a lot of sheep in Wales – and racking my brain to try and remember what they were called. Not their individual names but what the name for a sheep was. It was a

*Figure 4.2 PA Society Questionnaire – Chart showing **neurological symptoms** experienced by survey respondents (courtesy of the Pernicious Anaemia Society)*

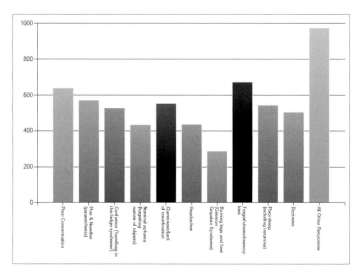

frightening experience that I kept to myself, but it happened often, which can be quite a problem when you are delivering a lecture to 50 professional adults and you forget the name of the subject you are talking about. Similarly, I remember watching the news on television and not being able to name the newsreader or, perhaps more worryingly, the name of the Prime Minister. It was all very disturbing, especially when you consider I hadn't heard of B_{12} deficiency and had no idea what pernicious anaemia was.

Another cognitive problem caused by pernicious anaemia is the confusion and absent-mindedness experienced by sufferers. This is described by members of the online focus groups as 'handbag in the fridge syndrome'. There is a special section on the online forum that deals with this issue – you'll find it in the Social Corner of the forum and it's labelled 'I know I need my jab when:...' Members explain what irrational things they have done when battling with the handbag in the fridge syndrome. These include:[ii]

ii These are original posts copied directly from the forum.

- Peanut butter in freezer; frozen waffles in fridge (frozen waffles so expensive; peanut butter doesn't require refrigeration).
- Finding Tuesday night's microwave pizza fully cooked but now cold in the microwave oven on Thursday.
- Finding the remote control for the garage door in the crisper drawer of the fridge, after paying for a new remote... best idea how this happened is that I eat apples a lot and got distracted... very expensive mistake.
- Starting to run a bubble bath, coming back two hours later to go pee and finding several inches of ice cold water on the floor (thanks/cheers for well-laid tiles as I was on the third floor and nothing leaked!!!)
- Unloading the dishwasher full of dirty dishes because I failed to put soap in before running it and/or I forget to start it (this happens frequently).
- [My personal favourite:] On carpool-to-work day, spending 45 minutes looking all over the parking lot for my Jeep, then checking the parking lot I never use, then asking security to notify the police. The police were halfway through filing the report before the friend I carpooled with found me in the main lobby in tears and pulled me aside to remind me that my Jeep was parked at his house (filing a false police report is $750 fine in CO and they probably only let me off because of my employer – they were very pissed off).
- I stare into space a lot; but, I know I need my injection when I am speaking and in the middle of a sentence I begin to stare off into space, then two seconds later I recover and finish my sentence. It's weird because my friends say it's as if I leave planet earth and go into another dimension but never acknowledge that I left (so they think, but I know I left).
- I know I need my jab... when I've marked 65 exam

papers to find out I've added all the numbers up … to scores which don't represent anything like the marks on the papers. Oops!

- Does anyone else get uber clumsy when it's time for their injection? I'm accident prone, scatty at the very best of times. But when my injection's due I seem to bump into everything, spill stuff everywhere and generally just mess up the simplest of tasks. This means that for the three weeks or so before my jabs I can't wear girly clothes as my legs are often so bruised that I look like I'm in an abusive relationship! (If anyone else gets this problem … buy spray-on tights, which are excellent at covering bruises !)
- It was my weekly washing day today so I stripped the bed down to the bottom sheet then collected towels and dirty clothes from the bathroom and piled them all onto the bed with the intention of making a big bundle and taking it all to the washing machine. Sometime later, I stood staring at the big pile of stuff on the bed and couldn't figure out what it was doing there.
- I forgot my own surname when we went to enrol our daughter for primary school. Oops. They looked very suspicious, especially as I'm very dark and she's very blonde. I also forgot the name for a bowl and had to describe it as 'that umbrella-shaped thing'. Gawd, it sounds even worse when it's written down.
- Walking around the kitchen asking for the 'pointy things' and making scissor shapes with my fingers...
- Saying, 'I want the thingy thing, have you seen it?'
- Leaving the dog at the supermarket, whilst carrying a 12-pack of dog food and stopping off to say 'hello' to another dog, then remembering I'd forgotten something, but not what. (I did go back and get her, but worst of all, it was all caught on the precinct's security cameras!)

- Turning up for various appointments either a week early or a week late.
- Putting the tea spoon in the bin and tea bag in the sink.
- Getting called 'dumm-bu' by my daughters' PE(!) teacher because I tuned out for her entire rant. (This one might have just been PE teacher syndrome...)
- Walking into a room 3-4 times because I only remember what I wanted when I go back to the original room I was in.
- Going into a shop, then forgetting what I wanted and staring blankly when the shop assistants ask if they can help me.
- Doing dodgy, possibly offensive and entirely unhelpful sign language to attempt to emulate what I want because I can't remember the word.

It is easy to dismiss the above as being the consequence of the stresses and strains of busy modern lifestyles and it could be argued that these occurrences can happen to anyone regardless of whether they have pernicious anaemia or B_{12} deficiency. Yet these are only a small selection of posts made by members of the Pernicious Anaemia Society who have taken the time to tell their stories. Anyway, if these sorts of things happen to apparently non-B_{12} deficient people, it doesn't mean they don't actually have a deficiency too; just because that person hasn't been diagnosed with pernicious anaemia or B_{12} deficiency doesn't mean that he or she isn't deficient – it could be that they just haven't been diagnosed – yet.

Peripheral nerve damage

Another set of serious symptoms of B_{12} deficiency manifest themselves in physical problems that can, if not addressed and treated, lead to the patient being confined to a wheelchair. Just as nerve damage can affect cognitive function, it can also have considerable impact on peripheral nerves – the nerves responsible for all nerve action outside the brain and spinal cord. The first sign of peripheral nerve damage is when the patient develops 'pins and needles' – known to doctors as 'paraesthesia'. The patient might also develop numbness, especially in the legs and feet; left untreated, this can lead to serious problems with walking and talking. In Chapter 1 of this book you read how I associated the numbness in my legs with the fall I took on that fateful night at the end of a gig. Over 18 months of visits to doctors, neurosurgeons and neurologists, not one of the medical professionals associated the numbness in my legs with B_{12} deficiency. I had MRI scans, and even the highly unpleasant Nerve Conduction Test, and yet nobody thought to check my blood. I can only begin to imagine just how many people throughout the world are having all kinds of physical problems that have not been associated with vitamin B_{12} deficiency. Today I still cannot run, and it's not a pleasant sight watching me trying to get up off the floor. And I make quite a sight descending stairs, although if there's nobody watching I descend backwards – I can go at quite a pace.

Swollen tongue

Another quite common symptom is a swollen and beefy tongue, although this isn't as common as is usually thought.[iii] This is often picked up by dentists, who can and do alert patients to their potentially having B_{12} deficiency.

Balance and co-ordination

There are other symptoms that are not automatically associated with pernicious anaemia and B_{12} deficiency that centre on balance and physical co-ordination. This is especially true if the deficiency has not been diagnosed for some time. Again, these symptoms are caused by nerve damage and they can manifest themselves to a greater or lesser extent.

iii Known as 'glossitis'.

The online focus group aptly named the particular balance problems found in B_{12} deficiency as 'the shoulder bumps'. The patient will often bump into walls, especially when descending stairs. Showering is particularly hazardous as one of the neurological problems involves not being able to stand upright with your eyes closed. Linked to this is another neurological symptom – vertigo, where, unless you have a visual reference point to compensate for any non-functioning balance mechanism in your brain, you become unsteady and dizzy. I cannot climb on a chair, let alone a ladder, and driving across bridges brings its own special challenges – I have just to concentrate on the number plate of the car in front.

Effects on behaviour

Another lesser-known group of symptoms concerns behaviour patterns. This is not, as far as I'm aware, mentioned in any medical textbooks, but it is these symptoms that have the greatest impact on family life and work. The full consequences of how B_{12} deficiency affects the patient's behaviour will be dealt with later (see page 173), but it is useful to list these symptoms here if only to help those living or working with a patient with pernicious anaemia understand how the condition can affect behaviour. They include:

- Mood swings, 'tear jags', heightened emotions;
- Irritability, frustration, impatience;
- A desire for isolation, quiet and peace;
- An aversion to bright lights and crowded spaces and, if these can't be avoided, the sufferer will become increasingly irritable and bad mannered.

These behavioural issues have only been identified, as far as I'm aware, by members of the Pernicious Anaemia Society and their families and friends. They are probably associated with not being able to handle everyday decision making and information input because of the impaired brain function caused by B_{12} deficiency.

And yet again, receiving replacement therapy injections of B_{12} doesn't mean an end to these behavioural problems in everyone. Obviously, these changes in behaviour patterns and sudden mood swings can lead to relationship breakdowns, work-related problems and friendship issues – again leading to the patient feeling isolated and depressed.

Newly identified symptoms and co-existing health problems

The time has come for the symptoms usually attributed to B_{12} deficiency to be thoroughly revised and updated so that existing and future doctors can be aware of their quite specific nature. In addition, there are symptoms – like the behaviour problems listed already – that are largely unrecognised by medical professionals, but clearly identified by members of the Pernicious Anaemia Society. There are a surprising number of these indicators of pernicious anaemia and B_{12} deficiency that are unknown to a great number of medical professionals. These symptoms have only emerged as pointers because members of the Pernicious Anaemia Society have identified them in their online postings on the forum and in telephone calls to the Society and to the Society's nurse counsellor.

- A burning sensation in the legs and or feet – this is called Grierson-Gopalan syndrome, and is caused by a lack of B_{12}.
- Brittle, flaky nails, often with ridges.
- Sudden unaccountable bouts of diarrhoea – often reported after a spell of constipation.[iv]
- Dry skin – anywhere on the patient's body.
- Insomnia – this is surprising considering that most patients could fall asleep on a washing line. This is a serious problem for those who suffer from it because, even

iv Dogs that have diarrhoea are treated using vitamin B_{12}.

*Figure 4.3 PA Society Questionnaire – Chart showing **emotional symptoms** experienced by survey respondents (courtesy of the Pernicious Anaemia Society)*

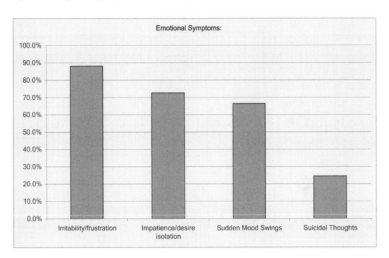

though the patient is exhausted, he or she cannot sleep for anything like the amount of time he or she would like. This, of course, leads to further frustration and irritation.

• Hair loss and premature greying.
• Arrhythmia – irregular, fast or slow heartbeat .

One of these symptoms – sudden, unexpected bouts of diarrhoea – is experienced by so many members of the Pernicious Anaemia Society that it is hard to believe it has not been identified by medical professionals as a strong indicator that the patient has either B_{12} deficiency or pernicious anaemia. It is the symptom most commonly experienced by members. As one member put it, 'It's more like anal incontinence than just diarrhoea. I didn't dare leave the house for days at a time.' This link between gastroenterology and B_{12} deficiency shouldn't come as a surprise when you understand that B_{12} absorption takes place in the small intestine – more of this later (see page 105).

The Society has also uncovered strong links between perni-

*Figure 4.4 PA Society Questionnaire – Chart showing **gastrointestinal symptoms** experienced by survey respondents (courtesy of the Pernicious Anaemia Society)*

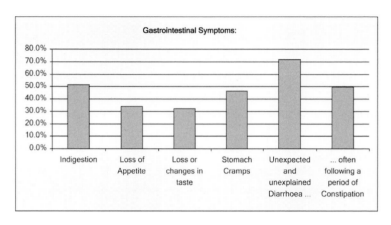

cious anaemia and other diseases (see Figure 4.5). It is apparent from the results of the survey, that if a patient is diagnosed with pernicious anaemia or B_{12} deficiency, it is highly unlikely that he or she will *only* suffer from the symptoms of that disease, but will most probably have one or more of the following conditions as well. These are listed in the order that they were experienced by respondents to the questionnaire, with the most 'popular' co-existing condition first.

- Tinnitus – ringing or screeching in one or both ears
- Hypo- or hyper-thyroidism – almost always, but not quite, experienced by females
- Fibromyalgia/neuropathic pain – often only on one side of the body
- Psoriasis
- Rosacea – a reddening of the nose and cheeks – sometimes referred to as the 'Curse of the Celts'
- Rheumatoid arthritis
- Vitiligo – white patches on the skin
- Myasthenia gravis – weak muscles leading to problems swallowing, chewing and opening your eye(s)

- Coeliac disease – intolerance to wheat and wheat products
- Psoriatic arthritis

Finally, one further strange condition has also been attributed to B_{12} deficiency – Lhermitte's sign, otherwise known as 'the barber chair phenomenon'. Patients with this syndrome will experience an electrical sensation running from their neck to their limbs. Lhermitte's sign is also associated with nitrous oxide abuse, which itself is responsible for destroying vitamin B_{12}. Very few doctors would make the association between what can be a very frightening condition and B_{12} deficiency and I am not aware it has been identified in any medical textbook.

Treatment does not resolve symptoms

As I have already described, but the textbooks do not say, the fourth major problem with the symptoms of B_{12} deficiency is that they do not necessarily disappear after treatment has begun. What

*Figure 4.5 PA Society Questionnaire – Chart showing the **co-existing conditions** reported by survey respondents (courtesy of the Pernicious Anaemia Society)*

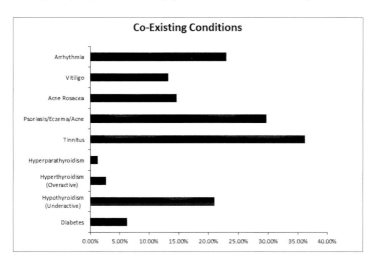

has become evident from the Pernicious Anaemia Society's log of telephone calls, letters, emails and online forum posts is that for the vast majority of the Society's members, replacement B_{12} therapy does not alleviate any or all of the symptoms described above. It is also evident that, in the past, when people complained about still experiencing the symptoms after their treatment had begun, doctors believed that the patient was imagining this – after all, there is no reason to suspect that the symptoms would still be present if a patient has a high or at least an adequate level of B_{12} in his or her blood. As it is the lack of B_{12} that led to the patient feeling unwell in the first place, why should he or she still be experiencing the symptoms once adequate treatment has started?

Before the formation of the Pernicious Anaemia Society, patients who complained to their doctors that their symptoms had not disappeared with the commencement of treatment were usually not taken seriously. Now, because there are simply so many members of the Society who do not find that the prescribed treatment makes their symptoms go away, this is being investigated. Similarly, a great many members find that they need far more frequent injections than those prescribed by their doctors – although why this is so has not, so far, been explained by medical professionals and will be discussed later on in the book (see page 85). Again, the sheer number of members of the Society who demand more injections than the number prescribed, means that this issue cannot be simply ignored.

Medical professionals are unable to offer any explanation as to why treated patients still have problems with thinking clearly and having normal memories after replacement therapy has begun. It could, as the haematologist surmised, be due to scarring of brain tissue owing to B_{12} deficiency in the past.

Patients who are refused more frequent injections than those prescribed by their doctors often source the injections from other places – with potentially dangerous outcomes. This will be discussed later on in the book (see page 144–146).

Conclusion

There are obviously, then, some serious issues with the symptoms of pernicious anaemia in particular, and B_{12} deficiency in general. The cost to health service providers throughout the world in not recognising them due to whatever cause must run into the billions of dollars every year. And the cost to individual patients and their families, friends and employers cannot be measured in money alone. The survey carried out by the Pernicious Anaemia Society indicates that there are a range of symptoms that doctors are not automatically associating with B_{12} deficiency, or pernicious anaemia in particular – and that is not because they choose not to do so or are being negligent; it's because until the Pernicious Anaemia Society was formed there was simply no organisation that could act as a focal point for patients' experiences. The original aim of the Society was to simply provide newly diagnosed patients with a clear and easy to understand explanation of the illness; unwittingly it uncovered serious problems with the way in which pernicious anaemia is diagnosed and treated.That is why the Pernicious Anaemia Society is campaigning for a thorough review of the way in which the symptoms of pernicious anaemia in particular and B_{12} deficiency in general are described to medical professionals. Only then will quick and accurate diagnoses be attained – to the benefit of the health service, the economy and the individual and his or her family and friends.

Unfortunately, reviewing and updating the symptoms of B_{12} deficiency will not, on its own, lead to an automatic improvement in the time it will take for patients to receive an accurate and timely diagnosis. That's because there appear also to be serious issues with the *way* in which B_{12} deficiency in general, and pernicious anaemia in particular, are diagnosed. It is to the diagnostic procedures that we shall now turn.

Poorly cats and dogs

During the filming of our documentary *Living with the Fog* we spoke to a stockman who worked on an organic farm. We were investigating claims made by some of our members that B_{12} was regularly given to cattle and we – that is, the documentary producer and I – were eager to find out more about this.

'Oh yes, we regularly give them shots of this,' said the stockman holding up a gallon jack of red liquid.

'Is it cyanocobalamin or hydroxocobalamin,' I asked rather stupidly.

'Oh, I don't know about that,' said the stockman. 'My Guvnor gets it from somewhere. He'd be the one to ask. Why don't I ask him to call you? He'd love to be in your film – he's always looking for publicity.'

I gave him my card that had the telephone number of the Pernicious Anaemia Society's office along with my mobile telephone number.

Back at the office, while waiting for the farmer to call, I began telephoning veterinary surgeons trying to get someone to speak to us about animals and B_{12}. Several told us that, if a dog or cat was brought to the surgery and the owner told them that whilst there was nothing obviously wrong with their pet, it was 'under the weather' and 'not him/herself', then the vets would inject the animal with B_{12} and that would generally result in the animal returning to normal. Not one vet would, however, tell this to camera. It is difficult to tell how widespread this practice is as another vet I spoke with told me that B_{12} would only be used in conjunction with other treatments.

The farmer never did call back although we tried to contact him on several occasions.

Chapter 5

Problems with diagnosing vitamin B$_{12}$ deficiency

This chapter explains how vitamin B$_{12}$ deficiency is diagnosed. We will examine the diagnostic pathway for pernicious anaemia in the next chapter – but here we will concentrate solely on vitamin B$_{12}$.

So how is vitamin B$_{12}$ deficiency diagnosed? Unfortunately, all too often it is not.

It begins with the patient, and here I would like to introduce you to Kay. As we have said before, one of the main characteristics of the symptoms of vitamin B$_{12}$, and pernicious anaemia, is that they are insidious and appear very gradually over what can be many years.

Kay is 39 years old with two children; one aged seven and one aged five. Kay has a busy life. She manages the home and has a full-time job working as a legal executive for a large firm of solicitors that specialise in property law. Kay began to feel tired two, maybe three years ago. Then the tiredness became mixed with exhaustion and lethargy. Kay began to spend longer at home and less time with her friends. The combination of constant tiredness, lethargy and fatigue led her to experience a strange tiredness which she had never heard of anyone else experiencing and she had not read about. Kay ignored these symptoms. She had a busy job where even more responsibilities had recently been given or, as she put it, 'dumped on her'. She had a husband and two children to care for – and lots of her friends said that they were tired too. And, of course, she was approaching middle age. She was bound to feel tired. She convinced herself that if she struggled through to the next summer, then two weeks in the sun would be all that she would need to feel herself again. Then other symptoms began to appear which she didn't associate with any particular illness. She started to forget things – everyday things. These were just silly little lapses at first, but they progressed to the stage where she couldn't remember the names of everyday items. 'Thingy' and 'what's its name' began to be used and heard more and more. Her family thought it hilarious. Then she began to experience recurring, unattributable bouts of diarrhoea at the same time as she began to have lapses in concentration at work, leading to warnings and threats. She doubled her efforts and began to go to bed earlier – much earlier than she was used to doing. Around this time she also became aware of a gradual ringing or screeching in her right ear before it also appeared in her left one. She started to become moody and irritable, which led to quarrels not only in her workplace but in the family home as well. She tried to relax by taking long hot baths, but all that produced was patches of dry skin. By two o'clock in the afternoon she was continually yawning and would stare at her computer screen and count the minutes before she could go home to bed. Kay was now finding it difficult to get up in the morning and, no matter how much sleep she had, would always wake up tired. The constant tiredness was beginning to make her feel down or even depressed and so she decided that she would visit her doctor. She was uneasy about going to see her GP, who had always been kind to her and who had the reputation of being a very good doctor. She hoped that she wasn't making a fool of herself, but her family and work colleagues' amusement at her behaviour was making her feel more and more down.

She eventually plucked up the courage to visit her doctor, who welcomed her into his room.

'What can I do for you?' he said in an extremely friendly way. Rather sheepishly Kay replied,

'I'm not feeling right. I am tired all the time, even if I sleep for 12 hours. And there's more; I keep forgetting the names of things, and

I'm irritable and moody. I do try to relax and I have lots of long hot baths but all that has done is to make me have dry skin. And I keep getting bouts of diarrhoea.' Kay didn't mention the fact that she was feeling depressed or the annoying ringing in her ears. She would take this one step at a time.

Now, in our first scenario what happens is that the doctor will be suspicious about Kay's tiredness and, after satisfying him or herself that Kay's lifestyle is not out of the ordinary, will order a full blood test and maybe ask that her thyroid be checked as well. Whether or not Kay's B_{12} levels and folate[i] will be checked will depend on a number of things. It will depend on whether the laboratory automatically carries out these tests anyway (but not all laboratories do this) or on whether the laboratory technician is prompted by the results of the other tests that are conducted in a full blood count to check Kay's B_{12} and folate. It could be that Kay's doctor asks for her B_{12} and folate to be checked alongside the full blood count. There is some evidence that many doctors will ask for this at the same time as the full blood count is conducted – but this doesn't happen in all cases.

In our second scenario, and in the real world, because the symptoms are vague, the doctor will just encourage Kay to take things easy, maybe take a holiday and see if things improve. Please note that I am not criticising GPs who offer this advice. Many patients who are feeling unwell may not even mention the continuing tiredness, which is the trigger that should alert the physician to investigate the patient's blood. As I have said, the symptoms are vague and will have developed over many years, so the patient may have learned to live with some of them long before and therefore simply won't even think to tell his or her doctor about them. I personally had advanced B_{12} deficiency that had already caused quite extensive nerve damage when I first

i Folate is the naturally occurring form of folic acid that is found in the body.

visited my doctor – but I didn't mention anything about how tired I felt.

In this second scenario, Kay will go home, maybe via a pharmacy where she may ask the pharmacist if he or she can recommend some kind of tonic that might alleviate the symptoms she is experiencing. Then she will relate what her doctor has said to her husband, who may mutter something about 'I told you so'. Kay will now feel isolated and alone. She will be reluctant to discuss how she feels with her friends and work colleagues because she will not want to sound as if she is continually moaning.

> Kay starts to stay at home. She has previously enjoyed going to the cinema one evening a week with her friends. She starts making excuses. Everything is becoming too much for her. She notices that she is waking up in the middle of the night with her heart pounding. She is hiding things at work – important documents that she is supposed to be dealing with and she pretends that she has never received them. She becomes more and more withdrawn. She eventually begins to wish she had never been born. Her symptoms are so vague, so attributable to other causes such as lifestyle, age, and the demands of modern family responsibilities, that nothing is being done – no investigations and consequently no treatment.
>
> Over the next year Kay's symptoms become more noticeable, but only slowly, gradually making themselves known. She now has no time for her husband, and her children are becoming a real burden. When her feet go numb and the pins and needles in her hands become almost unbearable she decides to visit her doctor one more time. She loses her balance as she walks into the surgery – previously she has only had problems with her balance when taking a shower. This time she is seen by a locum doctor who she has never seen before and who suggests that they might take a blood test – 'just to rule out any iron deficiency – we'll do a full blood count.'

A full blood count, or FBC, is a set of 10 separate tests that are carried out on a single blood sample and the results of these tests are interpreted by your doctor to give him or her a full picture of the health of your blood.[ii] As far as vitamin B_{12} deficiency is concerned, the important tests are those for haemoglobin, red blood cell count, and the red blood cells' 'mean corpuscular volume' (MCV). The MCV measures the size of the red blood cells and, if the cells are larger than they should be, then they are said to be 'macrocytic'. A lower than average amount of haemoglobin could suggest iron deficiency if the red blood cell count and the MCV are normal. However, if the haemoglobin count is low, as is the red blood cell count, with an elevated MCV, then that indicates B_{12} deficiency.[iii]

Long ago, doctors began analysing blood by taking a drop or two of the patient's blood and smearing it between two glass slides. The blood then becomes a film that can be analysed through a microscope. If the doctor knows what he or she is looking for, analysing blood film can be a valuable tool for doctors to make a diagnosis of many diseases. Things have moved on from individual doctors peering through microscopes to examine the blood film of a patient and nearly all FBCs are now carried out by complex and clever machines. Sometimes, most notably if the doctor is looking for evidence of childhood leukaemia, the blood is analysed manually by an individual using a microscope.

Whilst the FBC is undoubtedly a useful tool for helping doctors to make diagnoses, it should be noted that it doesn't include the test to measure the amount of B_{12} in the patient's blood. Either

ii White blood cell differential, haemoglobin, haematocrit, platelet count, mean platelet volume, mean corpuscular haemoglobin, mean corpuscular haemoglobin volume, red blood cell count, mean corpuscular volume, red cell distribution width.
iii I have simplified this for clarity. For iron deficiency, haemoglobin could be low or normal, the RBC could be low or normal, and the MCV could be low or normal. For B_{12} deficiency the haemoglobin could be low or normal as could the RBC and MCV. Are you now any clearer?

the doctor has to ask for the patient's B_{12} level to be measured in addition to, and at the same time as, the FBC, or, once the results have been examined and indicate that the patient might be B_{12} deficient, the patient will have to give up some more blood that will have its B_{12} status examined in a separate test. However, some analytical machines now automatically measure the level of B_{12} as well as carrying out the tests in the FBC. Sometimes levels of folate, or folic acid, are also measured.

If the analytical machine doesn't automatically measure the levels of B_{12} and folic acid in the blood, your doctor would have to ask for these tests separately. If he or she doesn't, the FBC only indicates the *possibility* that the patient has B_{12} deficiency. And the indicators of possible B_{12} deficiency are enlarged red blood cells (megaloblasts) and low levels of haemoglobin. However, there is a serious problem here. Low B_{12} levels do not always lead to the red blood cells becoming enlarged. Relying on the presence of mega-loblasts is dangerous because of the likelihood of the patient with low B_{12} levels, but no megaloblastic cells to indicate this, going on to develop serious and irreversible nerve damage.

To quote William Beck:

'Low serum cobalamin levels in the absence[iv] *of megaloblastic anemia is also encountered. In a study of 70 consecutive patients with pernicious anemia only 45 (64%) had very low cobalamin levels (i.e. under 100 pg/ml). Anemia was absent in 13 (19%) and macrocytosis was absent in 23 (33%).'[1]*

And according to Lindenbaum et al:

'Among 141 consecutive patients with neuro-psychiatric abnor-malities due to cobalamin deficiency, we found that 40 (28 per cent) had no anemia or macrocytosis.'[2]

iv My emphasis

So the FBC on which doctors rely so much will not necessarily identify potential B_{12} deficiency because the red blood cells may not be enlarged; as a result, even though the patient has the classic symptoms of B_{12} deficiency, he or she may remain untreated. As Carmel noted: 'The proscription that cobalamin deficiency should not be diagnosed unless megaloblastic changes are found is akin to requiring jaundice to diagnose liver disease.'[3]

This is further confounded by folic acid. Folic acid – or vitamin B_9 – prevents red blood cells becoming enlarged (macrocytic) and therefore further masks the sign of potential vitamin B_{12} deficiency. As Brouwer & Verhoef wrote: 'The study by Wyckoff and Ganji[4]... suggests that fortification with folic acid may have led to correction of macrocytosis, ie, increased mean corpuscular volume (MCV) of red blood cells caused by vitamin B-12 insufficiency.'[5] As a consequence, 'They (Wyckoff and Ganji) wisely concluded that MCV should not be used as a marker for vitamin B-12 insufficiency.'[6]

And folic acid further muddies the water because it can also reduce or mask the major symptom experienced by patients who are B_{12} deficient – the extreme tiredness. This will mean that the patient won't be able to provide the physician with one of the main indicators of B_{12} deficiency, thereby unwittingly delaying his or her own correct diagnosis.

Brouwer and Verhoef confirm this possibility: 'But what if the correction of macrocytosis is not only a doctor's problem, but is also a patient's problem? It is possible that the correction of anemia by consuming extra folic acid intake may not only correct the macrocytosis but may also lead to less fatigue among patients.'[7]

Folic acid was first identified in 1941 and was named after the Latin, *folium*, for leaf because it is found in abundance in leafy vegetables such as spinach, which contains 114 micrograms per 100 grams of the plant. Orange juice contains 90 micrograms, while breakfast cereals nearly all have folic acid added to them – Rice Krispies and Special K both have 330 micrograms per 100 grams.

These figures are dwarfed by the amount of folic acid in Ovaltine (400 micrograms) and yeast extracts such as Marmite (2,620 micrograms). These figures have to be taken in the context of the size of portions. An average portion of Marmite is around 4 grams (a medium-sized jar is 250 grams) whilst an average portion of breakfast cereal is 45 grams.

In North America, folic acid has been added to flour since the late 1990s to reduce the number of neural tube defects in babies. Neural tube defects (NTD) are the cause of spina bifida and other congenital conditions.

According to Grosse et al: 'In the US, Canada, Chile and Costa Rica, which all fortified flour between 1998 and 2000, the drop in NTD rates among live newborn babies was between 23 and 78 per cent.'[8] Currently no European country fortifies flour with folic acid, although there has been a healthy and lively debate about this going on for many years. The UK's Medical Research Council states on its website that the delay in fortifying flour with folic acid is because of the risk that B_{12} deficiency will be masked by the folic acid. 'This decision has been delayed due to a concern that folic acid fortification may harm people with undiagnosed vitamin B_{12} deficiency. This is because folic acid may eliminate the anaemia, which indicates B_{12} deficiency, but not the damage to the nerves, spinal cord or brain that lack of B_{12} causes.'[9] It then states that there is little evidence to support these concerns, which further muddies the debate.

What is certain is that large doses of folic acid are often routinely prescribed to pregnant women and sometimes to women who are trying to conceive; these folic acid supplements could mask the early signs of vitamin B_{12} deficiency.

Kay has just arrived at the nurse's room in her local surgery. For the past three months she has been buying a wide variety of vitamin supplements including folic acid. She dutifully rolls up her sleeve while the nurse takes several samples of her blood. The blood samples are placed in neatly labelled small plastic containers and are sent to the local hospital for analysis. If Kay's blood shows no enlarged red blood cells, then the laboratory's automated analyser will not highlight this in the test results. If Kay's haemoglobin is low, then the machine print-out will highlight this to the doctor who will then want to investigate the cause of the deficiency. Perhaps the laboratory technician will notice the low haemoglobin and will check Kay's ferritin level and hopefully her B_{12} levels. If these tests are not carried out, Kay's doctor will have to request them to find the cause of the low haemoglobin. But he may not and it has now taken two years or more for Kay to be given an explanation for her symptoms and a diagnosis.

There is a further problem with diagnosing B_{12} deficiency. Take a look at Figure 5.1, which shows how long members of the

*Figure 5.1 PA Society Questionnaire – Chart showing **how long it took respondents to receive a diagnosis** (courtesy of the Pernicious Anaemia Society)*

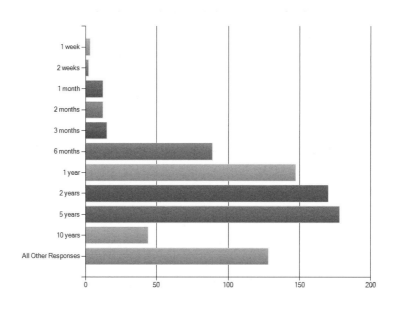

Pernicious Anaemia Society waited to be diagnosed eventually. Altogether, 26.3% went undiagnosed for five years, and 49% were undiagnosed for over two years. This is a serious issue because, left untreated, B_{12} deficiency leads to the patient developing serious nerve damage that is, in most cases, irreversible (see chapter 9).

By the time Kay's problem is diagnosed her family are no longer mocking her because she can't remember the names of everyday objects or because she is continually tired. What used to be thought of as funny has now developed into something very serious. She feels no better and now uses a walking stick to help steady herself when she shuffles about the house. She has had to stop working and only rarely can she rustle up the energy to venture to the local shops. Her hair has now started to fall out in handfuls and she has developed shooting pains from her neck into her right leg every so often when she bends her head forward.

Poor Kay, but let's take another scenario – a happier one. Let's assume that Kay's blood *does* show that she has enlarged red blood cells and her doctor immediately calls Kay and asks her to return to the nurse to give more blood so that he can investigate the cause which he suspects is low levels of vitamin B_{12}. This time the laboratory will test specifically for B_{12} concentrations and you would think that Kay will now be able to get a diagnosis. You'd be wrong.

The science behind how the amount of B_{12} in a patient's blood is measured need not concern us (which is me saying I really don't understand how they do it, although I have tried), but it is generally agreed that it is an accurate test to show how much of the vitamin is floating around in a patient's blood. The amount can be measured in different ways – otherwise it might seem far too straight forward a procedure! The laboratory results will either state the units of B_{12} in a patient's blood as being in picogrammes per millilitre of blood or in picomoles per litre of blood.[v] Picogrammes and picomoles are very small amounts and until as recently as 1979 the way in which the amount of B_{12} in a person's blood was calculated was unreliable. For the sake of simplicity I will stick with the picogrammes per millilitre method – pg/ml. And now we start to get involved in the real controversy surrounding the measuring of B_{12}.

Firstly, different laboratories will have different reference ranges for what are low, borderline and normal amounts of B_{12} in blood. This is because different laboratories use different machines, which have different reference ranges. You may ask yourself why don't all laboratories use the same make of machine and the answer involves, in Europe at least, anti-monopoly legislation. In the world of economics it would not be seen as good practice for one manufacturer to be the only provider of these complicated and highly technical analysing apparatuses. It may not make economic sense, but it would make the subject of test results much easier to understand. Anyway, different laboratories will have different reference ranges. And the printout that the machine produces, whoever manufactured it, will not only indicate the current status of the patient's blood but will also provide the number values of what that particular machine considers to be normal, borderline and low levels of B_{12} in the patient's blood – the machine's reference ranges.

Because different machines used to analyse the patient's blood will have different reference ranges, it is impossible to state with certainty what are normal, borderline and low figures. However, Pacholok & Stuart identified three common reference ranges that are used by different analysing machines to measure the amount of B_{12} in a patient's blood.

---

v You can convert from the former to the latter by multiplying by 0.738. The reason there are two types of unit is because originally chemical assays were expressed on a weight basis, and they still are in the USA. But in the 1960s an international agreement was reached that recommended expressing units in molar terms (i.e. related to molecular weight). It is called La Systeme Internationale (French spelling, SI).

The importance of testing for folate too

If a serum B_{12} test is requested, the patient's folate (naturally occurring folic acid) is not always automatically tested. But it should be: the Society's forum moderators have come to realise that there is a link between low folic acid and low serum B_{12} levels. What has become apparent is that members of the Society who report that their folic acid levels are low also report that their B_{12} levels haven't increased by any significant amount even after replacement therapy injections have been given. Yet, when advised by the moderators of the Society's online forum that they should also ask their doctor for folic acid supplements, and they take these, their B_{12} levels increase significantly. Why low levels of folic acid prevent B_{12} levels from rising is, as far as I'm aware, not common knowledge among medical professionals, but I have found a really important, but largely forgotten, research paper that explains this.[10] What this paper says is that if the folate status is low, the B_{12} in the patient's blood is low since much of the B_{12} will have been converted to forms of B_{12} that don't do what they should do – these are B_{12} analogues, which resemble proper B_{12} but they are not functional in the body nor are they detected by modern assay methods for B_{12}. What is clear is that folic acid levels have to be at concentrations that are normal or above for the replacement therapy of B_{12} to have any effect.

Typically the reference range might be:[11]

Less than 180 pg/ml	Low
180–350 pg/ml	Borderline
More than 350 pg/ml	Normal

What this means is that if your serum B_{12} result was 181 pg/ml, some interpreters would consider you *not* to be deficient in vitamin B_{12} but if your reading was 179 pg/ml you *would* be considered to be deficient. This strict interpretation of results causes much unhappiness and frustration among people who do not consequently receive any treatment even though they have all the symptoms of B_{12} deficiency. And this happens all too frequently.

These numeric ranges lead us to the second area of controversy in interpreting serum B_{12} results. In their book *Could It Be B₁₂? An Epidemic of Misdiagnosis* Pacholok and Stuart propose that, 'normal serum B_{12} levels should be greater than 550 pg/ml. For brain and nervous system health and prevention of disease in older adults, serum B_{12} levels should be maintained near or above 1,000 pg/ml.' The main reason they advocate this is because in the grey zone of somewhere between 180 and 350 pg/ml many patients present with all of the symptoms of pernicious anaemia but the physician is reluctant to begin treatment because the 'borderline' reading could be corrected by changes in diet. I know from telephone calls that I have taken in the Pernicious Anaemia Society office that doctors regularly send patients away when their B_{12} levels are in the grey zone, telling them to eat more red meat and come back in six months to be re-tested. 'Fair enough,' you might say; 'there's no need to treat someone if their levels *might* improve.' However, when you remember that the consequence of vitamin B_{12} deficiency is severe, irreversible nerve damage, then surely preventing B_{12} deficiency is the better option, especially as patients in this grey zone are often encountering problems at home, at work and in their social life? It doesn't make sense for a GP to suggest that the patient in front of them, whose serum B_{12} levels fall into the grey zone, should eat a more balanced diet – after all, their serum B_{12} was checked for a reason, most probably because they were displaying symptoms of B_{12} deficiency, and the FBC may even have revealed macrocytosis or low levels of haemoglobin.

People whose serum B_{12} levels fall into this grey zone are in a kind of no man's land.

You may ask yourself why the physician doesn't just prescribe B_{12} injections if the patient has some or all of the symptoms of B_{12} deficiency even if the test shows the patient's blood has B_{12} levels above the lower threshold? Remember, the injections are cheap, extremely safe and might improve the patient's wellbeing. Unfortunately, what usually happens is that the patient is not given the injections and he or she then makes repeated trips to the GP with the same symptoms, still asking for a diagnosis and treatment. The physician is left undecided as to the cause of the patient's symptoms because of the reliance on the test for serum B_{12}. I don't know how many times it is that I have taken a phone call at the office of the Pernicious Anaemia Society where the patient has told me that although he or she has all of the symptoms of B_{12} deficiency (usually they will have taken the 'Could You Be B_{12} Deficient Test' that is on the home page of the Society's website) their doctor won't prescribe them vitamin B_{12} injections because their reading is just one or two points above what the printout considers to be the threshold for B_{12} deficiency. This happens all of the time. As Pacholok and Stuart put it:

'Also, be aware that when it comes to B_{12} deficiency, many physicians tend to treat the paper laboratory report rather than the patient. Numerous times in our experience, a symptomatic patient's serum B_{12} was between 200 pg/ml and 300 pg/ml and the doctor told the patient, "You do not have a B_{12} deficiency". Given the remarkable safety of B_{12} treatment and the horrific *consequences of ignoring a deficiency, it is always best to err on the side of treatment.'[12]*

With so much criticism of the serum B_{12} test that is almost exclusively used to determine B_{12} deficiency, it is a wonder that it has survived in its current form and is still being used. This is, however, only half the problem. In the vast majority of cases that I am aware of, the results of the test are interpreted far too strictly. One of our members wrote to me telling me about her son's story. I have changed the name of the patient to preserve anonymity. I will quote the whole letter. I wish I could say this is an isolated case – but it isn't, and it is a continuous source of exasperation to me and fellow members of the Pernicious Anaemia Society.

'David. Age now 31. Close family history of pernicious anaemia.

'Recent B_{12} level at 252 in June 2011; cut off point for treatment at our surgery is 250. So he cannot be treated; the decision has been made by our doctor. David is, and has been, suffering from extreme tiredness and exhaustion plus many pernicious anaemia symptoms for most of his 31 years on this earth.

'I will start with David aged 5 weeks: operation for pyloric stenosis (stomach surgery) with many complications, including going into cardiac arrest after a serious internal haemorrhage 12 hours after the op. Always pale and tired. Slow to speak and learn, put down to deafness, grommets fitted, age 4 or 5.

'When he was about 7, David was repeatedly tired and run down; doctors thought he might have leukaemia. This was just before Christmas and we were told we would have to wait until after the New Year to find out, unless we went private, so we went private. This proved to be negative. I don't know what other tests were done at this time, but I would be very interested to know if B_{12} was included.

'David still remained pale, run down and unable to keep up at school. Educational psychologist appointed for David; the tests

showed he had an above average IQ. He was diagnosed with dyslexia, aged 8.

'David's feeling of not being the same, and not having the energy levels of his peers, affected his interaction with others. This is very sad as David is a kind and gentle person.

'Repeated visits to the doctors did not get us anywhere. In his teenage years David saw a consultant and was diagnosed with ME. Since becoming an adult, David has been labelled as having depression (yes, yet another label) and repeatedly given antidepressants, which he takes for a couple of months then stops, as he does not like the way they make him feel.

'Psychologically David has suffered tremendously. He becomes frustrated and angry with the exhaustion he suffers. Throughout his whole life he has been ridiculed and told he is lazy (to my shame I am, on occasion, guilty of this myself), he rarely goes to the doctors now because no one listens to him, and he thinks this is a waste of everyone's time. He pays well in his taxes and national insurance – yes, he has managed to hold down a job with immense difficulty. This though has been at a great cost to his social life. He comes home and usually goes to bed. He finds it extremely difficult to get up for work in the morning. At weekends he stays in bed, and it is quite normal for David to get up between 5 pm and 7 pm on his days off. He does not have relationships because this would involve using too much of his precious energy. Friends get bored with his constant lack of energy or enthusiasm, and his love of his bed. He is under weight for his height and looks very gaunt with a grey pallor.

'David has often walked into the lounge, flopped down and told me he feels like he is just "waiting to die". This is so heart breaking. David ticks almost all of the symptom boxes in your download.

'Where do we go from here????

'David has read the above and has agreed to allow me to forward this on to you.'

This is not an isolated case, and David's experience is one shared to a greater or lesser degree by thousands of others whose diagnosis and treatment are dictated by a test that should at the very least be viewed with a great deal of suspicion. His test result for serum B_{12} was 252 pg/ml and, although he had all of the symptoms of B_{12} deficiency, because his reading was above 250 he wasn't treated. Happily, David received treatment from another physician who realised the test is flawed and treated the symptoms rather than strictly interpreting the test results. He is now, according to his mother, 'a different man'.

There are those who are aware of the failings of the B_{12} test. Herrmann and Obeid state the following:

'Vitamin B_{12} deficiency is widespread. The neurological symptoms of vitamin B_{12} deficiency are unspecific and can be irreversible. Early detection is therefore important, using the most sensitive and specific markers available. Total serum vitamin B_{12} is a late, relatively insensitive and unspecific biomarker of deficiency.'[13]

I couldn't have put it any better myself so I'll let somebody else (Lee & Griffiths) do it for me:

'The clinical importance of a reliable human serum vitamin B_{12} assay to aid the diagnosis of pernicious anemia (PA) cannot be over-emphasized. Our review of the literature indicates that a reference method for the quantitation of serum vitamin B_{12} (serum B_{12}) with the required accuracy, precision and rapidity has not been reported to-date. Controversies, debates and criticisms over human serum B_{12} assays (especially commercial kits) have been commonplace.'[14]

There are other tests that can be used to detect B_{12} deficiency, but they are used only rarely. These include the methylmalonic acid test (MMA). Methylmalonic acid[vi] increases if the patient is deficient in B_{12}. Preferably the patient's urine should be analysed as it carries a far higher concentration of MMA than serum. Pacholok and Stuart state that the test is useful to rule out B_{12} deficiency while Herrmann and Obeid suggest that it could be useful if used in conjunction with the serum B_{12} test:

> 'Total vitamin B_{12} measurement is used cost effectively as the parameter of choice, but it has limited sensitivity and specificity, especially in persons with vitamin B_{12} concentrations < [less than] 400 pmol/l. If the total vitamin B_{12} concentration is in the lower reference range, 156 to 400 pmol/l, vitamin B_{12} deficiency cannot be ruled out.[vii] Clinical signs of vitamin B_{12} deficiency can be seen in persons with vitamin B_{12} concentrations within the reference range (> [more than]156 pmol/l). Persons with normal concentrations of vitamin B_{12} may have raised concentrations of MMA (>300 nmol/l).'[11]

In other words, MMA might be useful in determining B_{12} deficiency in a group of patients who would normally be deemed not to be deficient in B_{12}.

Another test for B_{12} deficiency is the test for the amino acid homocysteine,[viii] which is measured by analysing the patient's plasma. It too, like MMA, becomes elevated when the patient is deficient in vitamin B_{12}. Unfortunately, it also becomes elevated when there is a deficiency of B_6 and folic acid (B_9) and, as Pacholok and Stuart state, patients can have low homocysteine levels and be B_{12} deficient:

---

vi This is needed for fatty acid metabolism.

vii My emphasis – the problem is that people within this range (156-400) are, almost automatically ruled out of having B_{12} deficiency.

viii Amino acids are critical to life and play an important part in human metabolism.

'As with the MMA tests, we have seen many B_{12} deficient patients with normal Hcy[ix] levels who were symptomatic and either had a serum level less than 200 pg/ml or were in the grey zone.'[12]

And if you think we seem to be going around in circles here it's because we are. However, there's a new kid on the block of diagnostic tests for B_{12} that could be the answer to all of the uncertainties in diagnosing B_{12} deficiency that we have encountered so far. The new test differentiates between two types of B_{12} – and you thought it couldn't get any more complicated, didn't you? These two different forms of B_{12} come about because vitamin B_{12} in blood binds itself to two different types of protein. The two different proteins that 'marry' with the B_{12} (more correctly called cobalamin) are named 'transcobalamin' and 'haptocorrin'. When your cobalamin, or B_{12}, binds with the haptocorrin protein something strange happens – it doesn't do anything. It doesn't travel around trying to do anything biologically. Think of the bus analogy again. It will happily just amble by any bus-building projects and not get involved.

Any cobalamin that binds to the transcobalamin protein *will* make things happen; it will become biologically active and start making healthy red blood cells. The serum B_{12} test currently used doesn't differentiate between these two types of B_{12} – the 'active B_{12}' and the 'inactive B_{12}'.

Now we have to go back to the grey area of B_{12} levels where the amount of the vitamin in serum is between around 180 and 400 pg/ml or so. If a patient, who has all or some of the symptoms of B_{12} deficiency, has, say, a reading of total B_{12} of 350 pg/ml, then his or her doctor would not normally begin treatment because, as far as he or she is concerned, the patient would have B_{12} levels that are well above the deficiency threshold indicated by the test machine of, say, 200 pg/ml. The patient would remain untreated

---

ix The abbreviated form of homocysteine.

Figure 5.2 Proportion of active to inert vitamin B₁₂ in the circulation (Courtesy of Axis-Shield Diagnostics)

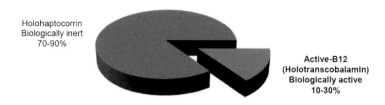

Holohaptocorrin
Biologically inert
70-90%

Active-B12
(Holotranscobalamin)
Biologically active
10-30%

whilst the doctor would spend time and energy on exploring other explanations for his/her symptoms.

But what if the patient had 50% of his or her B_{12} as the inactive kind, leaving only 50% of the B_{12} as active? The patient's true reading of biologically active B_{12} would be 175 pg/ml – way below the lower threshold indicated by the test machine readout. In fact, up to 90% of the B_{12} in your blood is inactive. (See Figure 5.2.) These figures have not been plucked out of thin air but are the result of very complex experiments that have been subject to strict quality controls to ensure their accuracy.

The main contributor to the discovery of active B_{12} was one of the most colourful characters in medicine in the 20th century, Victor Herbert. Herbert had the distinction of having served in four wars, the Second World War, the Korean War, Vietnam and Iraq.[15] As well as enjoying jumping out of serviceable aircraft, it was he who was responsible for instigating research into how this new form of B_{12} could be identified and counted. Along the way he also starved himself by eating vegetables that had been boiled many times in order to study the effects of folate deficiency.

His work has been developed into a test for active B_{12} by the multinational Axis-Shield, who produce all kinds of kits and equipment to help doctors to diagnose all manner of diseases. Given that there are so many problems with the serum B_{12} test that is currently used to diagnose B_{12} deficiency, this new test would mean that around twice as many people as currently would be diagnosed as being deficient in this crucial vitamin. Introducing the test would mean that patients would be diagnosed early and the 'grey area' of the serum B_{12} test would be eliminated as patients who are symptomatic, but with total serum B_{12} levels above the lower established threshold, would be diagnosed as being B_{12} deficient. This would mean that the repeated visits to the doctor to complain over and over about vague symptoms could become a thing of the past, thereby freeing up doctors' time. It would also mean that the main problem with the serum B_{12} test – that it is a late marker of B_{12} deficiency – would be eliminated and the risk of patients developing severe and irreversible nerve damage would be minimised.

Here's what Dr Murdo Black, the Director of R&D at Axis-Shield, has to say:

> 'The total serum B_{12} test, as the name suggests, measures all of the B_{12} in the circulation. However, not all of the circulating B_{12} can get from the blood into the cells of the body where it is needed for synthesis of DNA. Only holotranscobalamin, or active-B_{12}, can be taken up by cells and holotranscobalamin represents only 10-30% of the B_{12} in the blood. This means that the total B_{12} result can be misleading – a normal or even high total B_{12} result does not necessarily mean that you will have all of the B_{12} that your body needs. Typically, between 10% and 20% of samples with total serum B_{12} higher than the usual cut-off of 150 pmol/l could still be deficient according to the active-B_{12} result. The active-B_{12} result therefore represents a more accurate measure of a patient's true vitamin B_{12} status.'

On the downside, the new test is a little more expensive than the current test and it would mean that doctors would have to be trained to interpret the new test results. It would also mean that untold thousands of people would be told that they were deficient in B_{12} – even if they showed no symptoms. This could, of course, be seen as a good thing as it *prevents* symptoms developing rather than attempting to correct the product of B_{12} deficiency.

This new active B_{12} test seems to be the answer to all of the problems faced by many of the members of the Pernicious Anaemia Society. It would allow early diagnosis of B_{12} deficiency; it would solve the problem of patients being symptomatic but having B_{12} levels above the lower threshold used to determine deficiency (the grey zone); and it would improve the lives and wellbeing of thousands of people in the UK and millions throughout the world. The test is currently in use in a select number of laboratories and the scientific evidence for its reliability and accuracy have been rigorously examined.[16]

There is another test that has been developed and shows early promise. Researchers in Florida have used a breath test to determine whether a person has B_{12} deficiency.[x] They conclude: 'Overall, these results indicate that the vitamin B_{12} breath test is a noninvasive, sensitive, specific, and reproducible diagnostic test to detect vitamin B_{12} deficiency.'[17]

The only other way to improve the early identification of people with B_{12} deficiency would be to introduce Pacholok and Stuart's suggestion that:

'We believe that the "normal" serum B_{12} threshold needs to be raised from 200 pg/ml to at least 450 pg/ml because deficiencies begin to appear in the cerebral spinal fluid (CSF) below 550 pg/ml.'

… and

'At this time, we believe normal serum B_{12} levels should be greater than 550 pg/ml. For brain and nervous system health

x They estimate that 40% of Americans are suffering from B_{12} deficiency.

Chapter 5

and prevention of disease in older adults, serum B_{12} levels should be maintained near or above 1,000 pg/ml.'[12]

And there is hope that things might be moving in this direction. To quote Smith & Refsum:

'We believe that the traditional cut-off value of 148 pmol/l is too low. We suggest that physicians should consider treating patients who show symptoms but have vitamin B_{12} levels above this value, particularly those in the low–normal range up to ~300 pmol/l, in order to see whether their symptoms are relieved'.[18]

That's over double the threshold currently used to diagnose B_{12} deficiency.

Conclusion

This chapter has been concerned with the problems, and their possible solutions, that patients face in getting quickly and accurately diagnosed as having B_{12} deficiency. As there are so many issues surrounding the accuracy and reliability of the current serum B_{12} test it is a wonder that is still being used. What is certain is that the over-reliance by some, though not all, medical professionals on strict interpretation of test results to diagnose B_{12} deficiency affects individuals to varying degrees and impacts not only on patients' family lives, but also on careers and lifestyles. Introducing a much more rigorous procedure to determine early B_{12} deficiency would make economic as well as common sense, though perhaps doctors who don't bother to use the serum B_{12} test to diagnose deficiency but rely on the patient's symptoms are doing the right thing. And we could always follow the example of veterinary surgeons and farmers, who often diagnose animals with B_{12} deficiency and treat the animal without recourse to any blood test (see page 64).

87

When a patient *is* diagnosed as having B_{12} deficiency, the physician will often choose not to explore the cause of the patient's deficiency because, whatever the reason, the treatment will be the same. I don't have a problem with this because the current test to identify pernicious anaemia as the cause has its own problems. However, women of child-bearing age who have B_{12} deficiency and are considering having a baby *should* have the reason for their deficiency investigated. If the mother to be has 'intrinsic factor antibodies' (see chapter 6), then her baby will probably also have the antibodies as they can cross the placenta. A study from 1967 confirmed this:

> *'In the infant who had circulating intrinsic-factor antibodies, intrinsic factor could be detected at age 3 weeks in the gastric juice.'*[19]

The baby will then be in danger of also being unable to absorb vitamin B_{12} with all of the consequences. And, as we shall see, children with vitamin B_{12} deficiency probably caused by pernicious anaemia have their own set of problems to deal with.

In chapter 3 we discovered how difficult it would be to become deficient in B_{12} because it is present in a wide variety of foods and foodstuffs. We know that one of the causes of B_{12} deficiency is pernicious anaemia and we also know that many B_{12} deficient people do not test positive for that disease. Now there couldn't be a problem with the test for pernicious anaemia, could there? Well, we shall see (chapter 7), but first of all we need to know more about pernicious anaemia itself.

References

1   Beck WS. Neuropsychiatric consequences of cobalamin deficiency. *Advanced Institute of Medicine* 1991; 36: 33-56.
2   Lindenbaum J, Healton EB, et al. Neuropsychiatric disorders caused by cobalamin deficiency in the absence of anemia or macrocytosis.

New England Journal of Medicine 1988; 318(26): 1720-1728.

3   Carmel R. Current concepts in cobalamin deficiency. *Annual Review of Medicine* 2000; 51: 357-375.

4   Wyckoff KF, Ganji V. Proportion of individuals with low serum vitamin B-12 concentration without macrocytosis is higher in the post–folic acid fortification period than in the pre–folic acid fortification period. *American Journal of Clinical Nutrition* 2007; 86: 1187–1192.

5   Brouwer I, Verhoef P. Folic acid fortification: is masking vitamin B-12 deficiency what we should really worry about? *American Journal of Clinical Nutrition* 2007; 86(4): 897-898.

6   Ibid.

7   Ibid.

8   Grosse et al. Folic acid fortification and birth defects prevention: lessons from the Americas. *AgroFOOD industry hi-tech* 2006; 17: 50.

9   http://www.mrc.ac.uk/Achievementsimpact/Storiesofimpact/Folicacid/index.htm

10   Sheppard K, Ryrie D. Changes in serum levels of cobalamin and cobalamin analogues in folate deficiency. *Scandinavian Journal of Haematology* 1980; 25: 401–406.

11   Pacholok SM, Stuart JJ. *Could It Be B$_{12}$? An Epidemic of Misdiagnosis.* 2nd edition. Word Dancer Press, 2011.

12   Ibid.

13   Herrmann W, Obeid R. Causes and early diagnosis of vitamin B$_{12}$ deficiency. *Dtsch Arztebl Int* 2008; 105(40): 680-685: http://www.aerzteblatt.de/int/article.asp?id=61780

14   Lee DSC, Griffiths BW. Human serum vitamin B$_{12}$ assay methods – a review. *Clinical Biochemistry* 1985; 18(5): 261-266.

15   www.victorherbert.com

16   Obeid R, Herrmann W. Holotranscobalamin in laboratory diagnosis of cobalamin deficiency compared to total cobalamin and methylmalonic acid. *Clinical Chemistry and Laboratory Medicine* 2007; 45(12): 1746–1750.
     Valente E, Scott JM, Ueland PM, Cunningham C, Casey M, Molloy AM. Diagnostic accuracy of holotranscobalamin, methylmalonic acid, serum cobalamin, and other indicators of tissue vitamin B12 status in the elderly. *Clinical Chemistry* 2011; 57(6): 856-863.

17   Wagner DA, Schatz, Coston R, Curington C, Bolt D, Toskes PP. A new 13C breath test to detect vitamin B$_{12}$ deficiency: a prevalent and poorly diagnosed health problem. *Journal of Breath Research* 2011; 5: 046001.

18   Smith D, Refsum H. Do we need to reconsider the desirable blood level of vitamin B$_{12}$? *Journal of Internal Medicine* 2012; 271(2): 179–182.

19   Fisher JM, Taylor KB. Placental transfer of gastric antibodies. *The Lancet* 1967; 289 (7492): 695-698.

Vitamin B$_{12}$ and psychosis (2)

In 2000, Gary Payinda and Todd Hansen wrote in the *American Journal of Psychiatry* about one of their patients:

> *'Once the organic nature of her psychiatric illness was realized, the patient was given vitamin B$_{12}$ supplementation. Within two days the strength in her lower extremities had improved. Within two months her psychosis was completely resolved, and her only remaining deficit was unilateral weakness of the lower extremities and ataxia, although it was considerably less severe than when she was first seen. We can only assume that had her psychosis been recognized and treated as a symptom of vitamin B$_{12}$ deficiency much earlier, a complete reversal of her symptoms might have been expected.'*

Another episode relates to an 11-year-old girl who had been expelled from the Girl Guides because of her behaviour and who imagined that her school-friends were 'saying bad things' about her and planning to hurt her. She told one complete stranger that she could tell by his face that he hated her. Her doctor, R Denson, MD, reported in a letter to the editor of the *Canadian Medical Association Journal* in 1976 that:

> *'Because she refused to take any medication apart from vitamins, I prescribed vitamin B$_{12}$ in an easily ingested form, not expecting that it would influence the psychosis'.*

The cunning doctor planned to substitute the B$_{12}$ with more conventional drugs once the patient had become used to taking regular medication. However, the result of prescribing the harmless vitamin was:

> *'After she had taken crystalline vitamin B$_{12}$ (Redisol), 75µg for four weeks, the delusions and hallucinations had ceased. Her mother described the results of treatment as "amazing" and said, "It's like having a different child in the house. I used to dread her coming in but now it's a happy home." This striking improvement has been maintained for more than 12 months and vitamin B$_{12}$, 75 to 125 µg, is the only medication that has been administered. When the drug has been discontinued or the dosage much reduced, the parents have observed that the patient becomes moody and irritable within a few days.'*

Chapter 6

Pernicious anaemia, intrinsic factor and vitamin B₁₂

We have seen in the previous chapters that people may suffer from iron-deficiency anaemia because either they are not eating enough foods that contain iron, or they have experienced severe blood loss for one reason or another. Pernicious anaemia is different in that it is caused not by diet or by bleeding, but by the inability of the patient to absorb B_{12} from food. There are three causes of this problem and we will now examine these, but first a little about the history of the condition.

'Pernicious' is defined by the online Dictionary.com as: 'causing insidious harm or ruin; ruinous; injurious; hurtful, deadly; fatal: a pernicious disease'. It used to be the case that patients developing the disease would eventually, and after a long period of decline, die. This was because, until the second quarter of the 20th century, there was no effective or reliable treatment for the condition.

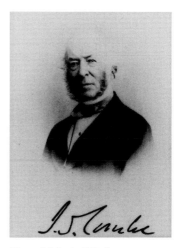

Figure 6.1 Portrait Dr James Scarth Combe (courtesy of Lothian Health Services Archive, Edinburgh University Library)

In the year 1824, the Edinburgh-based Dr James Scarth Combe had his first paper published in the *Transactions of the Medico-Chirurgical Society of Edinburgh*.[i] Entitled 'A history of a case of anemia',[1] Combe described a patient as having 'severe pallor, diarrhoea, extreme thirst and an excess of urine'. To medical professionals, 'pallor' indicates something more than just being off-colour. It is described by the *Oxford Concise Colour Dictionary of Medicine* as being 'an abnormal paleness of the skin, due to reduced blood flow or lack of normal pigment. Pallor may be associated with an indoor mode of life; it may also indicate shock, anaemia, cancer, or other diseases.' Whatever was the cause of this poor man's severe pallor it, and he, became the first case of anaemia to be reported in a medical journal. Dr Combe had identified the patient's pallor with something being wrong with his or her blood. And, what is more, he had used the word 'anaemia' for the first time in English, although it had been used by French doctors since 1761. The word itself is derived from the Greek *anaimia*, meaning 'lack of blood', from *an* 'without' and *haima* 'blood'. Incidentally the word wasn't used as an adjective – as in describing someone as being 'anaemic' - until 1840, and not until 1898 was it used in a figurative sense, as in 'this cup of tea is positively anaemic' – sorry, but that's the best I can come up with.[2]

Whilst the report published in the *Transactions of the Medico-Chirurgical Society of Edinburgh* didn't exactly set the medical world alight, it cannot have done the career of Dr Combe any harm as he became a Fellow of the Royal College of Surgeons of Edinburgh and he went on to become an Assessor for the College for many years, ending up as its President in 1851-2.[3]

In 1874, the *Medical Times and Gazette of London* published a letter by a German doctor, Anton Biermer, that described a new

---

i His second was published four years later in the *Edinburgh Medical and Surgical Journal* of 1828 entitled 'On the poisonous effects of the mussel (Mytius edlulis)'.

'idiopathic anaemia' that was not known in England.[4] This slur on the British medical profession was instantly countered by a certain Dr Samuel Wilkes who, within a week, had set the record straight in a letter to the *British Medical Journal* that stated that the disease *was* known in England, as Thomas Addison had lectured on it in 1843.[ii] Wilkes was a contemporary of Addison and was also a highly respected physician who was made Physician Extraordinary to Queen Victoria in 1897.[iii]

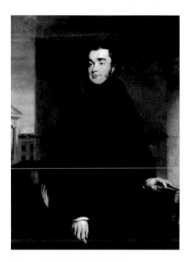

Thomas Addison's contribution to modern medicine is venerated in the Thomas Addison Unit of St George's Hospital London, in the Addison House Community Clinic Hospital in Harlow, and, no doubt in many other medical facilities. It is at Guy's Hospital in London, however,

Figure 6.2 Portrait of Dr Thomas Addison (reproduced by kind permission of the Gordon Museum, Kings' College London, and the Guy's and St Thomas' Charity)

that he is most remembered; a bust of him can be found in the Pathological Museum and a ward in the newest part of the building is named after him. A marble wall tablet can be seen

---

ii Biermer later lent his name to another title for pernicious anaemia – Addison-Biermer's disease. He also coined the term 'pernicious anaemia' in his 1872 work, *Über eine eigentümliche Form von progressiver, perniciöser Anaemi.*

iii Wilkes was the biographer of the 'Three Great' contemporary physicians who worked at Guy's Hospital: Dr Thomas Addison, the discoverer of Addison's disease, Dr Richard Bright, discoverer of Bright's disease, and Dr Thomas Hodgkin, discoverer of Hodgkin's lymphoma. He himself had discovered ulcerative colitis and his works were recognised when he was made a Baronet in 1898.

iv Not to be confused with Addison's disease – named after the same Thomas Addison, but which is a disease affecting the adrenal glands.

in the hospital chapel. It was Thomas Addison who is credited with identifying this particular disease, which is why pernicious anaemia is sometimes referred to as Addisonian anaemia.[iv]

Originally from Longbenton, near Newcastle upon Tyne, this remarkable doctor graduated in 1815, at the age of 21, with a degree in medicine from Edinburgh University, where he had enrolled just three years before. His thesis, which earned him his degree of Doctor of Medicine, was entitled 'Concerning Syphilis and Mercury' – although the full title was in Latin. (Addison was fluent in Latin – the language in which many medical texts were written at the time.) Two years later he began his career at Guy's Hospital, London, and by 1827 he was appointed Lecturer in *Materia Medica* – or, Medicine.

He was a hugely popular teacher, and it was during his time at Guy's Hospital in London that Addison built up his reputation as an expert in diagnosing all manner of diseases, often spending considerable amounts of time observing, examining and talking to patients in order to achieve a diagnosis. An introduction to a collection of his writings written by a third party gives us an insight into the intensity of his diagnostic probing:

> *'Possessing unusually vigorous perceptive powers, being shrewd and sagacious beyond the average of men, the patient before him was scanned with a penetrating glance from which few diseases could escape detection... [he] would remain at the bedside with a dogged determination to track down the disease to its very source for a period which often wearied his class and his attendant friends.'*[5]

Another example of his dedication to his patients and to ensuring that they were correctly diagnosed can be had from this quotation:

> *'Addison was at his best at the bedside, always moving to one side since he was slightly deaf in one ear. He used to tell his stu-*

*dents that if he could not reach a diagnosis in a patient he would
think of all the possible explanations for his patient's symptoms
on his way to and from the hospital. His abilities to sift evidence
and come up with a diagnosis were unrivalled in his day, but he
did not devote the same energies to alleviation or cure.'*[6]

Whilst Addison was an enthusiastic and talented diagnostician, the same, unfortunately, cannot be said of his approach to curing his patients. It seems that he put all of his knowledge and skills into producing a diagnosis and very little effort into treating the patients.

*'Once, when called in to see a patient he spent a long time in
finally arriving at the diagnosis of an abdominal cancer. He discussed this with the attending doctor and the patient's friends
and relatives and was leaving when he was reminded that he had
not written a prescription. He asked what he was already being
given and, when told "a magnesium mixture", he said "a very
good medicine; go on with it".'*[7]

It was at a lecture to the South London Medical Society in 1849 that Addison gave the first clinical and pathological description of 'this remarkable form of anaemia' which was later called 'Addisonian anaemia'[8] by a French doctor called Trousseau.[9] During the lecture, Addison described the symptoms, as observed by him, of this new type of anaemia:[v]

*'The countenance gets pale, the whites of the eyes become pearly, the
general frame flabby rather than wasted... the whole surface of the
body presents a blanched, smooth and waxy appearance; the lips,
gums, and tongue seem bloodless... extreme languor and faintness*

v I am unable to source the title of his talk but it can be reasonably assumed that it was the same as the title of the paper he published the same year – Chronics suprarenal insufficiency, usually due to tuberculosis of suprarenal capsule. *London Medical Gazette* 1849;43: 517-518.

supervene, breathlessness and palpitations being produced by the most trifling exertion or emotion; some slight oedema[vi] [swelling] is probably perceived in the ankles; the debility becomes extreme... the disease... resisted all remedial efforts and sooner or later terminated fatally... On examining the bodies I have failed to discover any organic lesion that could properly or reasonably be assigned as an adequate cause... .'[10]

Most or all of these symptoms will be recognised by patients with pernicious anaemia and their families and friends, although the reference to the tongue seeming 'bloodless' goes against what is seen as a sure sign of pernicious anaemia – namely, a swollen, red, 'beefy' tongue.

What is clear is that Addison correctly identified that the disease eventually results in extreme debility – 'the debility becomes extreme' – and finally the patient dies – 'the disease... resisted all remedial efforts and sooner or later terminated fatally'.

Addisonian anaemia, later to become known as pernicious anaemia, would continue to be diagnosed even though there was no scientific explanation for it. There were big questions that needed to be answered about why and how these patients displayed their symptoms, and the answers to these questions would take several decades to emerge.

In addition to Addisonian anaemia, Addison also identified Addison's disease, Addisonian crisis, and Addison-Schilder syndrome,[vii] yet he suffered from bouts of depression all his life and, in 1860, in a touching letter to the university authorities and his students, whom he evidently believed that he had let down, he took a career break in order to deal with his illness. His letter reads:

---

vi Swelling caused by fluid in the tissue.

vii He also made very important contributions to the identification of other diseases including Allibert's disease, Rayer's disease and Allgrove's syndrome.

'A considerable breakdown in my health has scared me from the anxieties, responsibilities and excitement of my profession; whether temporarily or permanently cannot yet be determined but, whatever may be the issue, be assured that nothing was better calculated to soothe me than the kind interest manifested by the pupils of Guy's Hospital during the many trying years devoted to that institution.'

He was 67 with evidently no intention of retiring yet. Three months later, on the 29th June 1860, he committed suicide despite being carefully watched by two attendants, who were aware that he had attempted to end his life before. The *Brighton Herald* reported on the following day:

'Dr Addison, formerly a physician to Guy's Hospital, committed suicide by jumping down the area [that is, the space between the front of the house and the street] of 15 Wellington Villas, where he had for some time been residing, under the care of two attendants, having before attempted self-destruction. He was 72 years of age [sic], and laboured under the form of insanity called melancholia, resulting from overwork of the brain. He was walking in the garden with his attendants, when he was summoned in to dinner. He made as if towards the front door, but suddenly threw himself over a dwarf-wall into the area – a distance of nine feet – and, falling on his head, the frontal bone was fractured, and death resulted at one o'clock yesterday morning.'

It was a sad end to the illustrious and productive career of one of medicine's truly great men.[11]

You may now be wondering why you are being given this history lesson about men, and, up until now, they have only been men, who have identified patients as suffering from some form of anaemia. The reason that Combe and later Addison deserve so much attention is that they first identified patients as suffering from a form of anaemia *without* the benefit of any examination of their patients' blood. Indeed, from the time that this disease was named Addisonian anaemia, at the beginning of the second half of the 19th century, until the first decade of the 20th century, doctors solely used observation of the symptoms to make a firm diagnosis because the science behind the diagnosis was simply not there. Combe and Addison compiled a set of reliable symptoms for diagnosing pernicious anaemia, even though they didn't understand the cause. Some observers of, and commentators on, the current diagnostic procedure would welcome a return to a diagnosis based on symptoms rather than what could be seen by some as the over-reliance on laboratory results to diagnose and treat patients with pernicious anaemia.

Whilst doctors following on from Addison's observations were now able to diagnose Addisonian anaemia, there was no treatment available, let alone a cure. It would be 100 years from the time Combe first described the condition to an effective treatment being made available.

In 1907, an American, Richard Clark Cabot, described 1,200 patients with pernicious anaemia who had a survival expectancy of between one and three years. Obviously this was a serious disease that was not being treated effectively and one that could strike any class of person – people whose diet was lacking in expensive meat were not the only ones who were vulnerable to the condition.

It was another American, William B Castle, who identified the all-important 'intrinsic factor' that is essential for the absorption of vitamin B_{12}. Dr Castle ran a quite ingenious, though particularly disgusting, experiment. He fed (via a tube into their stomachs) half of his patients suffering from pernicious anaemia, hamburger meat that he had eaten and then regurgitated an

viii He did this by 'pharyngeal stimulation' – sticking his fingers down his throat.

hour later.[viii] (Presumably he was good enough to feed them the regurgitated burger meat when it was still warm from the warmth of his stomach.) The other half of his hapless patients were fed un-regurgitated hamburger meat. The first group of patients responded to the 'treatment' while the second group did not. Obviously there was only so much hamburger meat that Dr Castle could regurgitate and the experiment could not be sustained, but it led the physician to conclude that there was something in a healthy person's stomach that worked on the meat to extract the goodness out of the food. (Vitamins hadn't yet been identified at this time.) Castle called this 'something' in the human stomach 'intrinsic factor'.[12] The 'extrinsic factor', in case you are wondering, was the food itself. The most amazing aspect of this experiment was that Castle didn't tell his patients what they were receiving; his explanations, if anyone asked, were masked in euphemisms and so not one of his patients knew that he or she was having regurgitated hamburger meat fed into their stomachs and they happily signed the consent forms.[13]

It wasn't until the 1970s that it was possible to identify and analyse intrinsic factor even though its existence had been known since the 1920s. And it is intrinsic factor, or rather a lack of it, that sets people with pernicious anaemia apart from others with other types of anaemia. A normal, healthy person will have in their stomach the protein called intrinsic factor. A person with pernicious anaemia will not.

An American, George Whipple, had an interest in all things to do with the liver and, quite by accident due to a laboratory technician not doing his job properly, found that giving liver to dogs who were anaemic hastened their recovery. Whipple had deliberately made the dogs anaemic by bleeding them, the consequence of which was that the dogs had only about a third of the amount of haemoglobin that healthy dogs had and were consequently lacking enough red blood cells to transport sufficient oxygen around their bodies. Whipple observed that the dogs fed liver recovered from their ordeal much more quickly than those fed other food. It has to be observed that, like Castle, he didn't explain clearly to his participants in the experiment exactly what he was doing – but the results were a major break-through in treating pernicious anaemia that led eventually to the 'pernicious' – that is, fatal – description of the disease becoming redundant.

The notion that liver could be used to treat pernicious anaemia was developed by two more Americans, George Minot and William Murphy, who discovered that liver juice was better than simple raw liver in keeping people with pernicious anaemia alive. They published their results in 1926, and in 1928 another giant in the history of American medicine, Edwin Cohn, managed to make a concentrate of 50-100 times the strength of liver juice, which meant that, providing the patient was diagnosed correctly, the pernicious part of pernicious anaemia became out-dated.[ix] In 1934, Whipple, Minot and Murphy shared the Nobel Prize for Physiology and their work led to the isolation of vitamin B_{12} in 1947 by Shorb, Folkers and Todd.[14]

By that year (1947) a highly concentrated form of liver juice had been available to doctors for nearly a decade to prevent patients diagnosed as having pernicious anaemia from dying. These preparations of concentrated liver were available from 1938 and I have a booklet produced by the Lily Corporation of America from that date that has advertisements for its 'highly concentrated anti pernicious anaemia principle derived from the liver'. The juice was injected into muscle every 10 days.

---

ix In his entry in Wikipedia it is noted that, 'Cohn would often give public demon-strations of the blood fractionation machine, in which he would fractionate his own blood on the stage during the lecture. In one such lecture, at the Instituto Superior Técnico in Lisbon, the machine became blocked (without Cohn's knowledge) and exploded, showering the first few rows of the audience with Cohn's blood. Cohn maintained his composure, however, and continued his lecture without significant interruption.'

During the 1950s, synthetic versions of vitamin B_{12} were developed by the research groups of Robert B Woodward and of Albert Eschemoser. It took a team of about 100 co-workers, working for over a decade, to perform the complete synthesis, thereby making liver juice concentrations that carried natural B_{12} redundant. Cyanocobalamin, and later hydroxocobalamin – the artificially produced B_{12} – began to be used to keep alive patients diagnosed with pernicious anaemia.

In 1956, Dorothy Crowfoot Hodgkin[x] identified the chemical structure of B_{12} (shown in Figure 6.3) for which she received the

Figure 6.3 The chemical structure of vitamin B_{12}, showing cobalt (Co) at its core (courtesy of Axis-Shield Diagnostics)

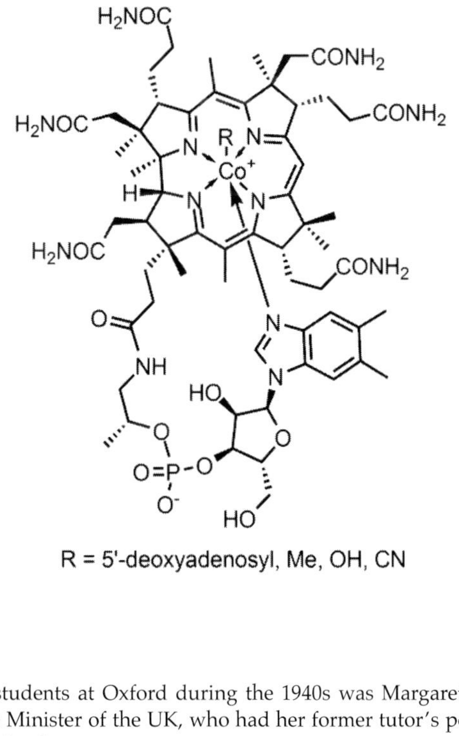

R = 5'-deoxyadenosyl, Me, OH, CN

x One of her students at Oxford during the 1940s was Margaret Thatcher, the future Prime Minister of the UK, who had her former tutor's portrait hung in No. 10 Downing Street.

Nobel Prize for Chemistry in 1964. This essential vitamin had, for a time, been the subject of choice for many of the greatest minds in medicine to investigate. It had taken scientists 100 years from Addison's observations to understand why people developed pernicious anaemia and how it could be treated. Finally, the importance and the characteristics of the vitamin B_{12} molecule were understood and its role in the correct metabolism of the human body appreciated.

As was noted at the start of this chapter, pernicious anaemia is different from iron-deficiency anaemia or diet-deficient anaemia because iron deficiency can be corrected by the patient eating iron-rich foods or taking iron tablets, while any diet deficiency can be corrected by the same methods. Patients with pernicious anaemia lack the intrinsic factor in their stomachs that is needed to extract vitamin B_{12} from any animal products – so no matter how good their diets, they will not be able to benefit from the B_{12} in their food. That's why pernicious anaemia is different from B_{12} deficiency – it's because of the lack of intrinsic factor. This leads to the next big question – why do some people lack this essential intrinsic factor?

It could be due to one of two things: either the patient isn't producing any intrinsic factor, or, bizarrely, the patient is producing the intrinsic factor but somehow simultaneously destroying it by also producing an antibody that will do so – known to doctors as the intrinsic factor antibody.

We need to know a little more about intrinsic factor to understand fully how lack of it can lead to pernicious anaemia. To do this we have to spend some time examining some more cells; this time it's 'parietal cells' that will be our subject, and they are to be found in your stomach.

The whole digestive process whereby all of the nutrients needed for a person to be healthy are extracted from food begins the moment you pop something edible into your mouth. As gin to chew the food and mix it with saliva, you begin the digestive process. Saliva is 98% water, but the other 2% is a rich mix of chemicals that include an enzyme and antibacterial agents. Chewing the food turns it into a 'bolus' – which is then swallowed and enters the stomach.

As mentioned above, there are parietal cells in your stomach – or at least there should be. The stomach's main function is to begin the process of food digestion, but your stomach is not the only organ that plays a part in this process. It provides just one stage in the digestive process (see Figure 6.4). The parietal cells in your stomach produce strong hydrochloric acid – the same innocent-looking colourless liquid that your chemistry teacher used to issue those dire warnings about. The acid is produced in your stomach to kill off any bacterial growth taking place in the food you have eaten before turning it – the bolus – into partially digested food called 'chyme'. The acid doesn't burn a hole right through you because of a mucous membrane that coats the stomach wall and judicious production of bicarbonate. If the mucous or bicarbonate fail to counter the acid, the result

Figure 6.4 The human digestive tract

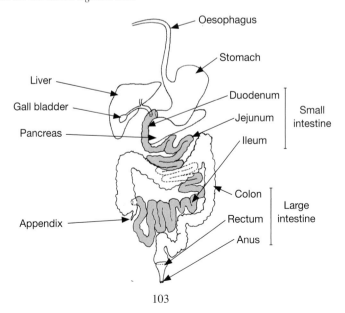

is heartburn and / or peptic ulcers. This is why people mix bicarbonate of soda (or sodium bicarbonate) with water and drink it to treat any acid indigestion that they might be experiencing. Antacids, such as 'Tums' neutralise acid that has already been produced. Proton pump inhibitors, which are among the most widely used medicines and include Omeprazole, Zanprol and Prilosec, are used to treat indigestion, heartburn and peptic ulcers among other things, and are so-called because they *inhibit* acid secretion. At the same time they may also inhibit the production of intrinsic factor.[xi]

The stomach also produces protein-digesting enzymes[xii] to aid food digestion at a later stage. So, contrary to popular belief, the stomach doesn't actually absorb any nutrients from the food; it simply turns the bolus – or chewed food – into a kind of soup by mixing it with acid and churning it into a pulp using smooth muscular contractions of the stomach wall. This chyme is then ready to be sent to the next stage of the digestive process. The length of time it takes to render chewed food into this soup depends on the type of food you have eaten and how well it has been chewed, but it can take anything between 40 minutes and a few hours.[xiii]

As well as producing an acid so strong that it easily dissolves iron and zinc, parietal cells also produce intrinsic factor – the mysterious substance first identified by Dr Castle, the great regurgitator.

---

xi Other medicines that interfere with B_{12} absorption are listed in the Appendix (see page xxx).

xii An enzyme is a substance that speeds up the process of a molecule being changed into a different molecule – as in food being changed into chyme. Enzymes are added to laundry detergents to make them 'biological'.

xiii Chewing food is important as it is the beginning of the process of efficient digestion. In 1903, a San Francisco art dealer called Horace Fletcher advocated chewing your food between 32 and 80 times until it becomes totally liquefied, and then spitting out what's left. Fletcher became known as the 'great masticator'. I can only begin to imagine how much fun his dinner parties were.

The intrinsic factor along with the partially digested foodstuff which, if you had eaten a piece of liver earlier, will also contain lots of vitamin B_{12}, then leaves your stomach for another piece of essential apparatus that you have had since you were born, the small intestine; this is where most of the food you eat is digested and the nutrients from the food are absorbed.

The small intestine is about 3 metres long and 1.5 to 2 centimetres wide – that is, around 10 feet long and an inch wide. The partially digested food is pushed into the small intestine by a muscle called the pylorus; it's all one-way traffic because the muscle is a sphincter muscle, the 'pyloric sphincter' – it allows the chyme in but won't let it out again. Because the chyme is highly acidic, the small intestine releases bicarbonate to neutralise the acid and then gets to work at extracting all the good stuff from the food. The chyme is broken down and all the nutrients extracted by 'digestive enzymes' (remember that enzymes are molecules that enable and speed up chemical reactions). These enzymes are produced by the pancreas – an organ that lies alongside the small intestine, and they enter the small intestine via the pancreatic duct.

There are three parts to the small intestine: the duodenum, the jejunum and the ileum (see Figure 6.4). Most of the nutrients in the chyme are absorbed in the jejunum, but there are exceptions. Iron is absorbed in the duodenum, and our friend vitamin B_{12} is absorbed in the ileum. And it's in the ileum that an amazing biochemical process takes place. The B_{12} binds with the intrinsic factor that was made by the parietal cells back in the stomach. The intrinsic factor/B_{12} compounds are recognised by special cells called receptors – ileum receptors – that line the walls of the ileum. Via some complex biochemistry, the intrinsic factor/B_{12} compound is absorbed into the bloodstream where, eventually, it will go on to help build healthy red blood cells.

There are other nutrients involved in some very complex biochemical processes that are beyond the scope of this book; basically, by a process known as diffusion, the digested food is converted into many different substances that enter the blood-stream and are carried to different organs of the body where they are used to build more complicated substances such as proteins that are vital to good health.

Any foodstuff that has not been digested is then passed onto the large intestine. The large intestine contains over 700 types of bacteria, known as gut flora, that create vitamins that find their way into the bloodstream. Various gases are also a by-product. Then, water is removed from any remaining foodstuff and it is prepared for eventual evacuation.[15]

In a rather gruesome experiment (that Hugo Minney describes on the www.b12d.org website), a professor at the Radcliffe Infirmary in Oxford, Sheila Callender, made a drink from people's own stools and demonstrated that it contained enough B_{12} to make up for any deficiency in the diet. In other words, firstly there are microbes in the human gut which are capable of making B_{12}, and secondly, that these microbes are too far along the gut for humans to absorb the B_{12} manufactured in this way. More recently, Professor John Hunter, who works at Addenbrooke's Hospital in Cambridge, has suggested that one cause of B_{12} deficiency is a rare situation where the microbes from the colon invade the ileum. Instead of manufacturing B_{12} for use by their human host, they grow rapidly and steal any B_{12} in the gut before the human can absorb it, leading to B_{12} deficiency.[16]

We noted that vitamin B_{12} is absorbed in the ileum and so it follows that if a person has had to have his or her ileum removed for whatever reason, then that person will be deficient in vitamin B_{12} and have to rely on injections of the vitamin in order to stay alive. One such person is Roy Sandford, from Fylde, near Blackpool. 'I had my ileum removed in 1989 and was told that I would need no other treatment once the wound had healed. I knew nothing about B_{12} and only found out how important it was when my GP was trying to find out why I was so tired all the time and why I couldn't concentrate. He decided to take some blood and discovered my B_{12}

levels were very low. Once I started treatment I felt so much better but it was the Pernicious Anaemia Society's website that alerted me to the fact that the current replacement therapy injection once every three months is hopelessly inadequate – I have now managed to convince my GP that I need the injection every month if I am to stop myself from experiencing all the awful symptoms again.'

This chapter has described the amazing journey that B_{12} makes from being sourced in foodstuffs to being absorbed into the bloodstream in a healthy person. If you are a healthy individual and eat a balanced diet that includes animal products, or you take dietary supplements including B_{12}, then you can leave it to the biochemical process that is continually at work in your body to produce adequate amounts of B_{12} to ensure that you produce healthy red blood cells that carry out their essential duty. There are, however, people whose biological function is impaired and who do not absorb vitamin B_{12} from food.

Some people produce organisms that destroy other organisms that their bodies have made. For example, some people produce parietal cell antibodies that effectively destroy the parietal cells responsible for producing the intrinsic factor that is needed to bind to B_{12} to allow it to be absorbed into the bloodstream. Then there are people who produce antibodies that destroy the intrinsic factor produced by their healthy parietal cells – intrinsic factor antibodies. Just why a person produces antibodies that kill off these essential elements that he or she has made in order to avoid dying is not known. There are other diseases that are caused by the body producing substances that attack essential substances and tissues that it has gone to the trouble of producing. For some unknown reason the body seems to think that what has been produced – in the case of pernicious anaemia either the parietal cells or the intrinsic factor – is an enemy (or pathogen) that has to be destroyed. These self-destructive diseases are known to doctors as 'autoimmune diseases' and they include Chrohn's disease, coeliac disease, diabetes mellitus type 1, Hashimoto's thyroiditis, psoriasis, psoriatic arthritis, rheumatoid arthritis and ulcerative colitis, to name just a few. The Pernicious Anaemia Society's survey shows that people with one autoimmune disease will almost always suffer from one or other of these other autoimmune diseases to some degree or other.

So – people with pernicious anaemia produce antibodies that destroy either their parietal cells or the intrinsic factor itself and, unless they can get B_{12} into their bloodstream by by-passing their digestive system, they will die. Before doctors found that liver could be used to treat pernicious anaemia, people diagnosed with the condition used to die a slow and unpleasant death; curiously they still do.

Nina Lawson was born in Scotland on 27th July 1926. She trained as a hairdresser in Glasgow and made a career in show business as a theatrical hairstylist. After working for the Sadler's Wells Opera and the Stratford Shakespeare Festival in Canada she took charge of the wig department of the Metropolitan Opera in New York City at the age of 30. She began purchasing, instead of renting, a vast collection of wigs and was highly respected by artists such as Birgit Nilsson, Luciano Pavarotti, Joan Sutherland and the young Plácido Domingo. It was said that never once did her immaculately groomed and pouffed wigs topple, no matter how vigorous the performance was being given by the most demanding of artists. Nina retired home to Scotland at the end of the 1986/87 season after 30 years in New York. Twenty-one years later, her obituary in the *New York Times* on 16th September 2008 informed her many admirers that she had died on 9th September 2008 aged 82: cause of death – pernicious anaemia.

I have been unable to determine why this lady died of a disease that had been treatable for over 60 years. It may be that she was undiagnosed and the cause of death was only determined at her post mortem. What is known, as we saw in the last chapter, is that there are serious problems with the way in which pernicious anaemia in particular, and B_{12} deficiency in general, are diagnosed.

Conclusion

It would be a good idea at this point to review what we have learned. Pernicious means ruinous, destructive and fatal. There are three possible causes of the condition: it can be due to lack of intrinsic factor because the parietal cells in the patient's stomach are not doing what they should be doing due to parietal cell antibodies attacking them; or the patient may have undergone surgery that has removed his or her ileum, which is the part of the intestines where the B_{12} passes into the bloodstream; or the patient may be producing, for some unknown reason, an antibody that neutralises his or her intrinsic factor. Any of these situations results in pernicious anaemia.

The first indicator of low B_{12} in the patient's blood is enlarged red blood cells, but we have seen that using macrocytosis as an indicator of low B_{12} is unreliable as people can and do have normal sized red blood cells yet be deficient in B_{12}. And we shall see that the only test now used to determine pernicious anaemia – the intrinsic factor antibody test – is unreliable. But what of the two groups of patients who do not produce any intrinsic factor – namely, those who have had their ileum removed or whose parietal cells, responsible for producing the intrinsic factor, are 'killed off' by parietal cell antibodies? They would not be producing any intrinsic factor and would test negative for intrinsic factor antibodies yet still have pernicious anaemia – they would be lacking B_{12}, which will eventually prove fatal if replacement B_{12} is not given. You guessed it – there are serious problems with diagnosing pernicious anaemia.

References

1   Combe JS. History of a case of anaemia. *Transcripts of the Medico-Chirurgical Society*, Edinburgh 1824; 1: 193-198.
2   http://www.etymonline.com
3   http://www.leithhistory.co.uk
4   I cannot find any original evidence of this letter but it is widely

reported and my source here is the Royal Society of Medicine's UKPubline Central.

5 Addison T. In: *A Collection of the Published Writings of the late Thomas Addison MD*. London: New Sydenham Society, 1868.

6 Whonamedit.com http://www.whonamedit.com/doctor.cfm/68.html

7 Ibid.

8 Ibid.

9 Sinclair L. Recognising, treating and understanding pernicious anaemia. *James Lind Library Bulletin: Commentaries on the history of treatment evaluation*. (www.jameslindlibrary.org) 2007.

10 Royal Society of Medicine's UKPubline Central (PMCID:PMC1079500)

11 From the Wikipedia article on Thomas Addison.

12 Castle WB. The effect of the administration to patients with pernicious anemia of beef muscle after incubation with normal human gastric juice. *American Journal of Medical Science* 1929; 178: 748-763.

13 Jandl JH. *William B Castle 1897—1990: A Biographical Memoir*. Washington DC: National Academies Press; 1995.

14 See individual entries in Wikipedia.

15 Callender ST, Spray GH. Latent pernicious anaemia. *British Journal of Haematology* 1962; 8: 230.

16 Hunter JO. *Inflammatory bowel disease: the essential guide to controlling Crohn's Disease, colitis and other IBDs*. London: Vermilion; 2010.

17 http://www.nytimes.com/2008/09/17/arts/music/17lawson.html

Chapter 7

Problems with diagnosing pernicious anaemia

In chapter 5 we examined the problems, and controversies with diagnosing vitamin B_{12} deficiency. When, and indeed if, a patient *is* diagnosed as having B_{12} deficiency, then most physicians would want to know the cause. I say 'most' because it turns out many members of the Pernicious Anaemia Society have not had an explanation for their B_{12} deficiency, as Figure 7.1 shows.

According to the Society's survey, 98.6% of its members have been told they are suffering from B_{12} deficiency, but only 79.5% have been formally diagnosed as having pernicious anaemia. For practical purposes, this isn't as big a problem as you might think. As long as the deficiency is being rectified with regular B_{12} injections, it makes little difference to patients if they have classic pernicious anaemia or not. There is a problem, however, if they want a firm diagnosis of the cause – there are serious difficulties with accurately diagnosing pernicious anaemia.

Now for an historical aside. On Thursday 21st November 1918, 10 days after the armistice, *HMS Cardiff*, a light cruiser that was less than a year old, was stationed in the North Sea. Following the orders of Admiral David Beatty, *Cardiff* led a fleet of 70 German warships into Scapa Flow in the Orkney Islands, which lie off the north east tip of Scotland. (The victorious allies were undecided about exactly what to do with the surrendered ships and the unarmed fleet was to be interred at Scapa Flow

Figure 7.1 PA Society Questionnaire – Chart showing what proportion of respondents had been diagnosed with (a) vitamin B_{12} deficiency, and (b) pernicious anaemia (courtesy of the Pernicious Anaemia Society)

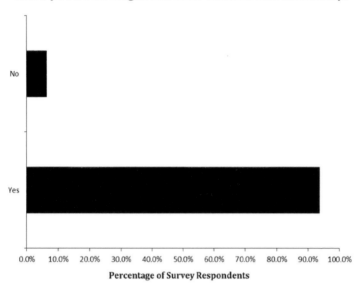

Have you been diagnosed with Vitamin B12 deficiency?

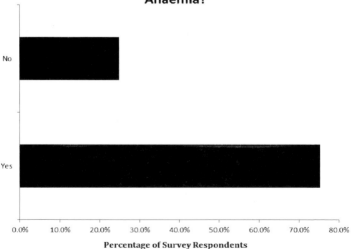

Have you been formally diagnosed with Pernicious Anaemia?

until a final decision was made. The following year, the Germans scuttled the fleet to prevent them being used by the victors.).

And that is how *HMS Cardiff* sailed into the history books. The light cruiser had a very uneventful life during the 1920s and '30s, and by the time the Second World

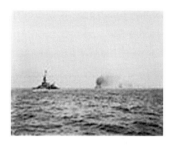

Figure 7.2 Photo of HMS Cardiff

War broke out she was almost obsolete, although she did play a part in the pursuit of the German battleships *Scharnhorst* and *Gneisenau*. In October 1940, she was withdrawn from operational service and spent the rest of the war as a training ship. In January 1946 she was sold and was broken up at Arnott Young breakers yard from 18th March of that year.

Now you will be perfectly justified in wondering what on earth does the brief history of a British light cruiser from the First World War have to do with diagnosing pernicious anaemia, so it will probably surprise you to know that it has a lot to do with 'nuclear medicine' in general and with getting an accurate diagnosis of the classic condition in particular.

I've been inside *HMS Cardiff* – the one that was broken up in Messrs Arnott and Young's yard; or rather, I've been inside a bit of her; it has been made into a special diagnostic room at Cardiff's University Hospital. And to fully understand why and how I ended up in part of a First World War cruiser we have to visit the world of steelmaking.

Steelmaking uses vast amounts of hot air, and in modern times that hot air is contaminated with radioactive material. The hot air used is not any different from the air that you and I are breathing right now, and so, yes, you are breathing radioactive air, but it's not as contaminated as it once was. Before 1963, when the Atmospheric Test Ban Treaty was signed, the world's atomic powers detonated 502 nuclear devices with the equivalent force of 440 million tons of TNT. And these were all conducted at sites above the ground, which meant that there was an awful lot of radioactive air around. These tests were in addition to the two atomic bombs dropped on Japan at the end of the Second World War.[1] Since 1963 the air quality has improved, although disasters at Chernobyl, and more recently at Fukushima, have ensured that the air surrounding us continues to contain radioactive material. Whether the amount of this radioactivity is harmful or not is still being hotly debated and I'll leave it at that.

What is certain is that any steel produced after 1945 will contain some radioactivity because the enormous amount of hot air used in its manufacture will inevitably have been radioactive. Now, if you want to measure how radioactive a person is you would have to ensure that none of the materials used in the experiment, including steel, was in any way radioactive and so the steel would have to have been manufactured *before* 1945. You may now be starting to make the connection with *HMS Cardiff* but it is likely you are also wondering why you might want to measure how radioactive a person is.

During the latter half of the 20th century, a new branch of medicine developed – nuclear medicine. Of all the branches of medicine, this one must surely have the scariest name. Think nuclear, and Chernobyl, Three Mile Island and Fukushima spring to mind – nuclear and medicine don't immediately appear to be happy bedfellows. The reassuring news is that the amounts of radioactivity used in nuclear medicine are tiny and are strictly controlled. The specially built room in Cardiff's University Hospital, using steel from *HMS Cardiff* is used to conduct a variety of tests using nuclear medicine. (There are, of course, many other such rooms around the world, but the Cardiff one is a special place for me.) And the reason why we are examining nuclear medicine is because it is by using radioactive substances that pernicious anaemia can be diagnosed with some degree of certainty.

A person eating a normal, healthy diet will be able to source enough vitamin B_{12} from his/her food to produce healthy red blood cells. As we saw in chapter 5, if a person has a healthy diet yet doesn't absorb B_{12} then that is most likely to be due to him or her either not producing any intrinsic factor or producing antibodies that 'kill off' the intrinsic factor. For around 50 years, until early this century, one way in which doctors could determine whether a patient was absorbing B_{12} would be to give him or her an injection of B_{12} that would saturate the areas in the body where B_{12} is stored – mainly the liver. Then, once the tissues were saturated, the patient would be given radioactive B_{12} to eat or drink. The radioactive B_{12} would be considered 'excess' and would be excreted by the patient in his or her urine as there would be no spare capacity in which to store it. (When a patient receives an intravenous infusion of B_{12} via an intravenous drip the urine turns the colour of a very good rosé wine because of the excess B_{12} being excreted.) Because the patient had swallowed excess radioactive B_{12} you could use his or her urine to determine whether or not he or she was actually absorbing B_{12} by testing to see if the urine was radioactive. That is because B_{12} can only get into the urine by combining with intrinsic factor and being absorbed in the ileum; otherwise it just stays in the gut and is egested along with all the other matter the body can't digest.

If less than 7% of the radioactive B_{12} was detected in the patient's urine, then he or she would undergo another test where he or she would swallow some intrinsic factor and then, after a little time, some more radioactive B_{12}. If the patient's urine then had more than 7% of the radioactive B_{12} in it, he or she could confidently apply for membership of the Pernicious Anaemia Society (except that it didn't exist then!), because he or she would definitely have had pernicious anaemia. The test would demonstrate that only after being given intrinsic factor could the patient absorb the B_{12}, showing that he or she was not producing intrinsic factor him/herself.

This test was named after the doctor who developed it – Dr Robert Frederick Schilling of the University of Wisconsin.

Dr Schilling developed it in the 1950s and, although it was not anywhere near 100% accurate, it was used to allow doctors to make a firm diagnosis of pernicious anaemia. However, it was expensive and time-consuming, and when the radioactive isotope that was used in the test became hard to source, it gradually stopped being used, in the early years of this century.

I don't think I ever had the Schilling test performed; I can't remember in those foggy days during which I was diagnosed ever being asked for a urine sample. But I did have a 'whole body count', which is where the total amount of radioactivity in my body was measured, once before I had swallowed some radioactive B_{12}, and then after I had taken the B_{12}. I remember I had two sessions, with the second session involving radioactive intrinsic factor. It was a completely painless procedure that involved a scanner passing around my body – but as I said previously, it was just after being diagnosed and so it was all a blur. I believe I am one of only a few members of the Pernicious Anaemia Society to have undergone this procedure, but it did allow my doctor to be confident in asserting I had full-blown, or 'classic', pernicious anaemia.

So, if the Schilling test is no longer available, what test is used to confirm a doctor's suspicion that a patient has pernicious anaemia? Well, there's the test that is used to determine if the patient is producing the antibodies that destroy intrinsic factor, the **intrinsic factor antibody test**. But there are serious concerns about the accuracy of that test. Here's what a reputable Australian study said about the test for intrinsic factor antibodies:

> '*A negative intrinsic factor antibody result does not exclude the diagnosis of pernicious anaemia as only 60% of patients with pernicious anaemia will have this antibody.*'[2]

Then there is the **parietal cell antibody test**. This can reveal if a patient is producing antibodies that destroy the parietal cells which are responsible for producing the intrinsic factor in the first place. But this is unreliable because its accuracy depends on the age of the patient being tested (see the quotation below where being under or over 50 years changes the interpretation of results). In fact, there are so many 'ifs' and 'buts' that interpreting these tests is very complicated. Here's what the Australasian Society of Clinical Immunology and Allergy, in conjunction with the Royal Australasian College of Pathologists, has to say about these tests in their *Consensus Guidelines on Anti-Intrinsic Factor Antibody Testing* from 2004. This is a direct quotation of the actual words used; as you will see, these are often difficult to follow:

> **'If both parietal cell antibody and intrinsic factor antibody are positive –**
>
> *[that means] immunological evidence of pernicious anaemia*
>
> **'If both parietal cell antibody and intrinsic factor antibody are negative –**
>
> *[that means] no immunological evidence of pernicious anaemia*
>
> **'If parietal cell antibody is positive but intrinsic factor antibody is negative –**
>
> *'Gastric parietal cell antibody is associated with >90% of patients with autoimmune gastritis, the end result of which may be pernicious anemia (PA). In 20-30% of patients, relatives of patients with PA, autoimmune thyroiditis and a small percentage of healthy persons may be positive and run an increased long term risk of pernicious anemia. A negative intrinsic factor antibody result does not exclude the diagnosis of pernicious anaemia as only 60% of patients with PA will have this antibody.*
>
> **'If parietal cell antibody is negative but intrinsic factor antibody is positive –**
>
> *[that means] immunological evidence of pernicious anaemia (if the patient has low Hb macrocytosis and low B_{12} levels)*
>
> **or** *(if only low B_{12})*
>
> *'The clinical significance of these results is uncertain in the absence of anemia or macrocytosis. Suggest repeating in 6*

months with serum gastrin, full blood count and fasting B$_{12}$.

'If parietal cell antibody is negative but intrinsic factor antibody is positive –

(if >50 yrs old)

[this means] immunological evidence of pernicious anaemia

(if <50 yrs old)

Suggest confirmation of diagnosis of pernicious anemia with gastric biopsy.

'If intrinsic factor antibody is positive and parietal cell antibody not done –

(if >50 yrs old)

[that means] immunological evidence of pernicious anaemia

(if <50 yrs old)

Suggest testing for gastric parietal cell antibody to confirm diagnosis of pernicious anemia.

'If intrinsic factor antibody is negative and parietal cell antibody is not done –

Suggest testing for gastric parietal cell antibody (GPC) because intrinsic factor antibodies (IFA) are found only in about 60% of patients with pernicious anemia (PA) whereas GPC is an excellent marker for autoimmune gastritis associated with pernicious anemia.

'If parietal cell antibody is positive and intrinsic factor antibody is not done –

Gastric parietal cell antibody is associated with >90% of patients with autoimmune gastritis, the end result of which may be pernicious anemia (PA). 20-30% of relatives of patients with PA, autoimmune thyroiditis and a small percentage of patients may be positive and never reach the stage of PA. If PA is suspected, we suggest testing for antibodies to intrinsic factor.'[3]

See what I mean? I tested negative for the intrinsic factor antibody twice before finally testing positive. I think it may be because of this that I was sent to that special little room at the

University of Wales Hospital in Cardiff, where the tests confirmed that I did indeed have classic, full-blown pernicious anaemia.

It's worth mentioning here that people with gastric atrophy[i] (sometimes caused by the bacterium *helicobacter pylori*) will not be producing any intrinsic factor either yet would test negative for intrinsic factor antibody. Consequently, they wouldn't be diagnosed as having pernicious anaemia, even though they would certainly have anaemia that is pernicious unless they received replacement B_{12} in the form of injections. And as we have already seen, if a patient has had his or her ileum removed they might be producing intrinsic factor but it wouldn't be doing what it is supposed to be doing, which is to bind to B_{12} and enter the bloodstream via the ileum.

B_{12} deficiency in people who do not have pernicious anaemia

Type 'B_{12} deficiency' into an internet search engine and you will get some idea of how much debate is currently going on about the subject. There is even a dedicated organisation in the North East of England that campaigns to get B_{12} deficiency more widely recognised.[ii] Debates rage on websites set up by clinicians and other medical professions about how widespread B_{12} deficiency is. And then there is Facebook, where over 20 groups, or pages, concern themselves with B_{12} in some form, although some of the pages are hosted by companies selling B_{12} products and there is one page for a group of musicians who have formed a musical group called 'B_{12}' and who play alternative musical instruments – with the result that the music is very alternative indeed. Why

i Also known as atrophic gastritis. Gastric atrophy is caused by long term inflammation of the mucous in the stomach leading to impairment in producing the essential substances needed for digesting food, including intrinsic factor and hydrochloric acid.
ii www.b12d.org

are so many people experiencing the symptoms of B_{12} deficiency and yet do not have pernicious anaemia?

There are two main reasons. Firstly, if their serum B_{12} is above the lower threshold for clinical B_{12} deficiency, their doctors will not consider them to be B_{12} deficient even though they may be experiencing and presenting all of the classic signs of the condition. And because they are not considered deficient, they will not be tested for intrinsic factor antibodies. In other words, they probably have pernicious anaemia but haven't been tested for it. Secondly, as we have seen, there are serious problems with the tests being used to give a definitive diagnosis of pernicious anaemia.

If a person is eating a healthy diet, and yet is experiencing the symptoms of B_{12} deficiency, then there has to be a reason for this – and it is my belief that there are many thousands of people, perhaps millions worldwide, who have pernicious anaemia but whose B_{12} levels are above the lower threshold used to categorise them as being B_{12} deficient and so who are not tested for pernicious anaemia. Alternatively, they have tested negative for intrinsic factor antibodies and so have been told they do not have pernicious anaemia. There has to be a reason for the deficiency, and the reference range and the test do not seem to be doing what they should be doing to find this out.

Of course, raising the lower threshold for determining B_{12} deficiency, as advocated by Professors Smith and Refsum, and Sally Pacholok and Jeffrey Stuart (see pages 76–78), would lead to a great many additional people being tested to discover the cause of their deficiency – and it might even lead to the diagnosis of pernicious anaemia in some or all of those people. And let's not forget the problem of the current serum B_{12} test that is in use, which only identifies the *total* amount of B_{12} in a patient's blood and does not distinguish between the biologically 'active' B_{12} and the biologically 'inactive' B_{12} that we discussed in chapter 5. If that test was introduced, almost certainly more people would be shown to have B_{12} deficiency and would need to be investigated to uncover the true cause of their deficiency, leading to many more people being diagnosed as having pernicious anaemia.

Because there is no definitive test for the condition, and because the current tests are notoriously inaccurate, one important positive indicator of pernicious anaemia is a family history of the disease. Whilst writing this book I was continually asked what would be the title of the work. One that I toyed with for quite a long time, and which was at one point its working title, was 'My Gran Had That'. This was because when I tell people that I have pernicious anaemia, a common response is, 'Oh, my Gran had that', usually followed by, 'She used to have really painful injections.' I don't mention that if their gran had the disease, then it is likely that they will also develop it, but perhaps I should. If I do mention it, I inevitably end up running through the whole list of symptoms that can indicate the disease – and as those symptoms are so vague and associated not only with other diseases but could be the result of a modern lifestyle, it is not very productive.

Pernicious anaemia runs in families. This has been understood by doctors for decades and there is some evidence that, in the past, doctors would consider a family history of the disease as being a solid indicator for a positive diagnosis. Someone who has investigated the genetics of pernicious anaemia is Dr Siddharth Banka. Dr Banka has recently finished a preliminary study into whether pernicious anaemia does indeed run in families. I asked him what his studies have shown thus far and how he plans to take his findings further. His reply is quite remarkable:

'We have shown that if your sibling has pernicious anaemia, then in comparison with the general population, you are more than 40 times more likely to develop B_{12} deficiency. We have also identified a number of families where pernicious anaemia runs from one generation to another. Overall, this means that it's a highly heritable condition and genes play an important role in determining pernicious anaemia susceptibility.'

On the down side, if you are reading this and one of your close family members has pernicious anaemia, there's a good chance that you will also develop the disease. On the plus side of course, at least you have a good indicator of what your symptoms are caused by. What is certain is that much more research needs to be conducted into the genetics of pernicious anaemia and Dr Banka seems determined to continue his work.[4]

'Large-scale genetic studies are expensive and time consuming. Our data show that genetic studies in pernicious anaemia, such as the one we are undertaking, are likely to be very successful. Increasingly, genetics is illuminating our understanding of diseases and thus providing opportunities for targeted and personalized management. As many patients with pernicious anaemia also suffer from other autoimmune diseases like diabetes and hypothyroidism, understanding pernicious anaemia genetics has scope to reveal pathways that may be important to a large number of patients.'

Another problem associated with diagnosing pernicious anaemia is the mistaken belief, not only among the public but also within the medical profession, that the condition mainly affects elderly women and only rarely is it to be found in men and younger people. This is not what the Pernicious Anaemia Society's survey showed. The survey asked members to state their age when they were diagnosed as having pernicious anaemia. The results are shown in Figure 7.3.

Patients visiting their doctor with all the signs and symptoms of B_{12} deficiency, which, if their diet is not an issue, is probably caused by pernicious anaemia, will not usually be associated with the disease if they are in an age group that medical professionals erroneously believe to be very low risk for the condition. And whilst it is true that as a person gets older and leaves middle age behind, he or she risks developing pernicious anaemia caused by gastric atrophy that can be attributed directly to ageing, Figure

7.3 shows that over 50% of members of the Pernicious Anaemia Society were diagnosed during their 30s or 40s.

The problem of misdiagnosing pernicious anaemia

Just a few minutes spent reading the stories of members of the Pernicious Anaemia Society on the online forum will lead you to understand just how widespread the problem of misdiagnosis is. Figure 7.4 shows the results of a further question in the Society's survey: 'Were you diagnosed as having another disease before being diagnosed with pernicious anaemia?' The detail of members' responses was hugely varied but analysing this shows that depression is the most common misdiagnosis, with irritable bowel syndrome coming second, and there is a wide range of other illnesses from anxiety to multiple sclerosis

Figure 7.3 PA Society Questionnaire – Chart showing the age at which respondents were diagnosed as having pernicious anaemia (courtesy of the Pernicious Anaemia Society)

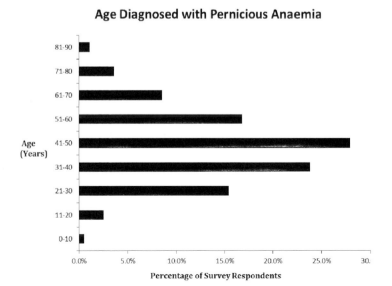

123

that members have originally been diagnosed with. The cost of repeated visits to doctors in trying to get an accurate diagnosis and subsequent treatment is difficult to estimate – but it is bound to be significant.

You should by now be getting the picture – B_{12} deficiency is a major problem and tests for diagnosing pernicious anaemia as the cause are unreliable and badly need investigating. And this problem manifests itself in two ways. Firstly, it leads to patients waiting a long time to receive a diagnosis – see the chart in chapter 5. Secondly, it means that physicians are not doing a very good job through no fault of their own. This in turn leads to patients feeling frustrated, angry and let down by the medical professions. Take a look at the chart in Figure 10.1 (see page 171) from the question in the Society's survey: 'How do you rate your medical care?'.

Add together all of those in the survey who believed the way in which their condition was investigated and diagnosed was 'very poor', 'poor', 'unreasonable' or 'inadequate', and you arrive at a staggering 52.9% of people who believe their experience was at the least inadequate and at the worst very poor. On the other

Figure 7.4   PA Society Questionnaire – Chart showing the proportion of respondents who were misdiagnosed with another condition before being diagnosed with pernicious anaemia (courtesy of the Pernicious Anaemia Society)

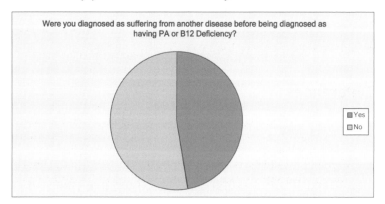

hand, 20.6% thought the way in which they were investigated and diagnosed was good or very good, with 3.3% classing their experience as excellent.

Conclusion

There is no cure for pernicious anaemia, and as far as I'm aware, nobody is currently searching for one. Instead, patients who are diagnosed with the condition have to rely on injections of B_{12} as replacement therapy – for life.

It is impossible to determine how many people have pernicious anaemia because of the unreliable diagnostic tests. A great many people have B_{12} deficiency but fall into the grey zone of what David Smith and Helga Refsum call 'sub-clinical cobalamin deficiency',[5] and because they do, will not have the cause of their deficiency confirmed with a robust diagnosis. As noted in chapter 5, the problem could be because of other medications that they are taking, but it could also be because they have pernicious anaemia. It won't be until their serum B_{12} levels fall below the current (far too low) threshold that is used to classify someone as having B_{12} deficiency that the cause of the deficiency will be examined, using tests that are unreliable. In short, the whole issue of B_{12} deficiency and pernicious anaemia is in a mess and nobody, at the time of writing, appears to be doing anything about it. And this confusion with diagnosing B_{12} deficiency and pernicious anaemia is having profound effects on people's lives. It is these consequences that we will now examine.

References

1   http://www.straightdope.com/columns/read/2971/is-steel-from-scuttled-german-warships-valuable-because-it-isn-t-contaminated-with-radioactivity This reference contains further references.
2   Consensus Guidelines on Anti-Intrinsic Factor Antibody Testing: Australasian Society of Clinical Immunology and Allergy in conjunc-

tion with the Royal Australasian College of Pathologists. 1 Nov 2004. http://www.allergy.org.au/images/stories/pospapers/ASCIA_Guidelines_IFA_1-%20Nov04.pdf

3   Ibid.

4   Banka S, Ryan K, Thomson W, Newman WG. Pernicious anaemia – genetic insights. *Autoimmunity Reviews* 2011; 10: 455–459.

5   Smith D, Refsum H. Do we need to reconsider the desirable blood level of vitamin B_{12}? *Journal of Internal Medicine* 2012; 271(2): 179–182.

The lucky horse

I have a private number plate. It comprises the letter B followed by the number 12 and then the initial letters of my name – B12 MVH. It was cheap and I treated myself to it for my 50th birthday. I was at a service station one day when the owner came out to talk to me and laughed at my number plate. I explained that I had pernicious anaemia and needed regular injections of B_{12} and that the other letters were my initials.

'I've got loads of B_{12} at home,' he told me.

'Oh!' I said. 'Do you have pernicious anaemia?' He laughed again.

'No, no, no. I give it to my horses.'

'Your horses?'

'Yes. I have three racehorses. We regularly give them decent shots of B_{12}.' 'Why do you give your racehorse B_{12}?' I asked, genuinely surprised and curious.

'Well,' he hesitated. 'Let's just say it makes them more compliant.'

I remember relating this incident to some of the members of the Pernicious Anaemia Society at a social event. One of the members told me that she used to work for a racehorse syndicate and they would often inject one particular horse with B_{12} and then travel around the area placing medium sized bets on the horse so as not to arouse any suspicion. The horse would invariably win the race.

Chapter 8

Treating pernicious anaemia

The previous chapters have described the problems with diagnosing B_{12} deficiency in general and pernicious anaemia in particular. As we've seen, these problems are responsible for a great many patients waiting a long time, sometimes many years, to receive an accurate diagnosis of what is causing their symptoms. Once a definitive diagnosis has been given you would assume that the patient's troubles would be over and that he or she would be able to correct the B_{12} deficiency quickly and easily. This assumption would, however, be wrong.

There are two things that need to be made clear before we embark on our investigation into how pernicious anaemia is treated. Firstly, most patients with the condition continue to experience the symptoms even after treatment has been started. For some, the symptoms are experienced to the same extent as they were before replacement B_{12} therapy began. Others find the injections alleviate some of the symptoms a little, whilst a further group find that their symptoms almost disappear. Nobody knows why this is as, theoretically, the symptoms should disappear completely. Secondly, the current treatment regimes that are provided by mainstream healthcare providers in different countries (see Table 8.1 later in this chapter) are suited to some patients, but not all. I've met people in the UK who manage perfectly well on the standard treatment – one intramuscular injection of B_{12}, in the form of 1 mg/ml hydroxocobalamin, every three months. These patients do not tend to join the Pernicious Anaemia Society because..., well, because they don't need the information and peer support that the charity provides to still symptomatic members. The vast majority of members of the Society do not manage well on the current mainstream treatment. And this causes all manner of problems.

The treatment of pernicious anaemia is by far the most frequent cause of complaint by members of the Pernicious Anaemia Society. These complaints come in many forms, via the telephone, letters, emails, and postings on the online forum. We record the subject matter of telephone calls to the office, and calls about inadequate treatment are so common that we – that is, myself and the other volunteers who staff the Society's offices – refer to them as 'the usual thing'.

One week in July 2011, the volunteers who run the Pernicious Anaemia Society kept a record of the subject matter of 20 successive telephone calls to the Society's office. Of these, one was a wrong number,[i] one was from a member informing us of a change of address and 18 were requests for information about how to get more frequent injections of vitamin B_{12}. In other words, nine out of 10 telephone calls that we received were enquiries as to how the caller could get more frequent injections. This little experiment just confirmed what we already knew – that the treatment of pernicious anaemia is the subject that causes by far the greatest frustration and anger among sufferers and it leads to many patients treating themselves without the knowledge or consent of their doctors. It also causes health inequality.

Usually it is the patient him/herself that calls or writes to query their treatment but sometimes a family member will make

i A window-blind manufacturer has our telephone number on their website for some reason.

the enquiry because they have noticed behavioural changes in their loved one in the run-up to the next injection. On average the Society gets three telephone calls a day regarding the current treatment regime and it is the number one topic on the Society's online forum.

I remember my own experience (see chapter 1). I found I was unable to manage on the normally prescribed treatment regime in the UK. Only when I went to see a second haematologist was I allowed injections 'on demand'. When I asked him why I needed more frequent injections his reply was, 'We don't know, but there are so many of you who feel they need more frequent treatment, we have to listen to you.' I was lucky. And I was lucky that my GP listened to the haematologist as I have discovered that, contrary to popular belief, GPs do not always follow the advice, or even instructions, of hospital consultants.

Healthcare should not be subject to luck, yet there are a whole series of barriers that stand in the way of a person receiving replacement therapy injections based on his or her individual needs, and overcoming these does seem to depend very much on luck. I shall try to explain these barriers as clearly as I can. And while I do so, you have to remember that the injections are life-savers for people with pernicious anaemia as there is as yet no cure for the condition.

Old-fashioned treatments

The discovery by Minot and Murphy in 1926 that patients with Addisonian anaemia could be kept alive by feeding them large quantities of raw liver meant that patients with pernicious anaemia no longer inevitably died of the condition, although their quality of life would vary greatly. Minot and Murphy's discovery led the Harvard-based Edwin Cohn to produce concentrated liver juice, which began to replace a liver-rich diet as the recommended method of treating pernicious anaemia. A book,[1] called *The Anemias* (with no acknowledged author), published in 1938, not only contains information for patients about the nature of the disease but also has 10 different daily diets that all contain liver in some form. Alluringly, towards the end of the book are advertisements for injections of liver extract. So it seems that for two decades, until the introduction of B_{12} injections in the form of cobalamin, liver-rich diets co-existed with the new liver extract injections. The introduction to the section on 'Diet in the Anemias' begins:

> *'The following section on "Diet in the Anemias" is partly of historical interest inasmuch as the present trend is toward instruction of the patient to eat a normal diet and depend upon parenteral injections of liver extract or oral administration of a suitable preparation of concentrated liver to control his anemia.'*

The idea, pre liver extract injections, was that the patient ate as much liver as he or she could in the hope that some of it would be converted into B_{12} – even though he or she might not have any intrinsic factor. And if you have bad memories of school lunches containing liver that was overcooked and dry, then the patient on a liver diet would probably be very envious of you. As the book says:

> *'The meat in the diet should be served rare without the addition of fat. It is best for the patient to eat raw liver. If he cannot do this, plain broiled liver should be served (200 grams per day). Some people can eat liver better if onions or tomatoes are added.'*

If I had the choice of raw or overcooked liver I know which one I would go for.

Here are the menus for one day given in the book, which I would imagine would turn mealtimes into something to dread rather than to look forward to:

BREAKFAST	GRAMS	AMOUNT
Grapefruit juice	205	1 cup
Broiled chicken liver	100	4" x 6½"
Whole wheat toast	30	1 slice
Butter	10	1 pat
Tea or coffee		
Sugar	4	1 teaspoonful
Cream	12	1 tablespoonful

LUNCHEON		
Tomato juice	205	1 cup
Liver sandwich on	100	1 large serving
whole wheat bread	60	
Buttered cauliflower	100	¾ cup
Milk	240	1 cup
Stuffed prune salad		
with cottage cheese	50	3 prunes
Fresh fruit cup	100	2/3 cup

DINNER		
Bouillon	200	1 cup
Wafers	10	2
Roast lamb	100	1 large serving
Kale	100	1 cup
Scalloped potatoes	180	2/3 cup
Whole wheat bread	30	1 slice
Butter	10	1 pat
Waldorf salad	100	½ cup
Date pudding	80	½ cup
Tea or coffee		
Cream	12	1 tablespoonful
Sugar	4	1 teaspoonful

There are also instructions on how to prepare 'liver drink', which is made using raw liver and grape juice, though it does say that:

'Tomato or orange juice may be substituted for the grape juice. The grape juice seems to disguise the liver taste better than the other juices.'

Then there's 'liver pulp' and 'creamed liver soup (two

servings)'. (I can't help thinking that these two portions were both for the patient rather than an extra portion for a healthy adult who didn't have to eat a soup made from raw liver and milk.) 'Tomato stuffed with liver' also contains raw liver while the recipe for 'scalloped liver' concedes that the reader may 'parboil liver'. You'd have to prepare the delightful sounding 'liver loaf' to get any cooked liver.

As the book was produced by a pharmaceutical company that was advertising its liver extract injections I cannot help thinking that they might have deliberately chosen unappealing menus. However, the recipes are based on the recommendations of Minot and Murphy, who were the first to recognise the benefits of feeding patients raw liver. If I was to follow these diets, I don't think it would be long before I would be succumbing to the lure of the advertisements for liver extract injections.

When Folkers and Todd identified cobalamin in 1948 and labelled their discovery 'B_{12}', the stage was set for an even more effective treatment for pernicious anaemia, and by the early 1950s artificial B_{12} was being produced in injectable form and the market for raw offal took a nosedive. Over the following years, several different forms of B_{12} injection began to be produced.

Current treatment

The current treatment regime in the UK, as already noted at the start of this chapter, is one 1 ml intramuscular injection of 1 mg/ ml hydroxocobalamin, every three months. As I will describe in greater detail (see page 134), replacement B_{12} is available in three main forms: cobalamin, hydroxocobalamin and methylcobalamin, with different countries favouring different forms (see Table 8.1). Each has its own pros and cons, but the most important point that will emerge from this account is that different patients have different needs, and any one-size-fits-all regime is inevitably going to fail some patients. Flexibility is needed and if the healthcare system does not provide that flexibility patients are often forced to take matters into their own hands – if they have the means.

Why injections?

The first point to consider is why patients with pernicious anaemia need to receive injections instead of taking B_{12} supplements orally in the way millions of people throughout the world do every day. The reason is, of course (if you have been following what I have been saying in all the previous chapters), that a patient with full-blown, or 'classic', pernicious anaemia will lack the intrinsic factor in his or her stomach that would normally bind with available B_{12} and allow it to enter the bloodstream. By injecting B_{12} directly into the bloodstream, the patient can by-pass the complex biological process that a healthy person would be able to rely on to get his or her B_{12}. One piece of research[2] has shown that patients diagnosed with pernicious anaemia could be treated using tablets of very highly concentrated B_{12}, but most patients, and doctors, prefer to treat the condition using injections.

People who have the symptoms of B_{12} deficiency and who have a serum B_{12} level that falls within the 'grey zone' (see page 77) but have not tested positive for intrinsic factor antibodies (and are therefore thought not to have pernicious anaemia), are also treated by injection even though they could also in theory swallow tablets to rectify any deficiency. Interestingly, such patients report that the injections seem to work while swallowing a tablet of B_{12} doesn't. I believe that this is not imagined or psychological but is because the intrinsic factor antibody test is so unreliable. These patients with low B_{12} probably do have pernicious anaemia, but the test hasn't managed to identify the intrinsic factor antibody – why else would they want to receive what can be painful injections?

Why on prescription?

The second point to address is why it is not possible to buy injections of B_{12} 'over the counter' at pharmacists. Why is it that the injections are available only on prescription in many countries, including the UK? The reason for this in the UK is the Medicine Act of 1968, which defined three types of medicines: those that are available only from a pharmacist with a prescription written by a physician – Prescription Only Medicines, or POMs; those available from a pharmacy – known as Pharmacy Medicines or PMs; and those medicines, such as aspirin, which are widely available in retail outlets – those on the General Sales List, or GSLs.

Now you may wonder why a harmless but essential vitamin is only available if the patient can persuade his or her physician to write a prescription for it, when potentially much more dangerous medicines can be bought in supermarkets. The reason is that it is an injection. In the UK, anything that is injected can be obtained only via a prescription from a doctor.

This in itself should not be a problem. Doctors write millions of prescriptions every year and just because B_{12} is one of these medicines it shouldn't be a problem – but it is. It's a very big problem because of the guidance doctors are expected to follow in writing prescriptions for B_{12}. And this is replicated in many other countries around the world.

As noted before, there are three types of B_{12} injection on offer. In some countries more than one is available, though most countries only use one. The three available forms of cobalamin (B_{12}) are cyanocobalamin, hydroxocobalamin and methylcobalamin. (There is a further type, called adenosylcobalamin, but as we have previously seen it is not produced in any large quantity because it is very unstable.)

Cyanocobalamin is the most widely used type. Hydroxocobalamin is, however, favoured by some countries (including the UK – see Table 8.1) because it is supposed to be retained by the body for longer. It is usually, with only rare exceptions, prescribed to be injected once every three months, while cyanocobalamin is generally administered, in countries where it is available, once a month. The three-monthly regime has the advantage of reducing the number of times patients need to be injected; injections can be painful, but more importantly to the NHS and its equivalents, while the B_{12} is inexpensive, health professionals' time is not. The evidence that hydroxocobalamin is retained for longer is, however, extremely weak. Here's what researchers who compared cyanocobalamin with hydroxocobalamin found in 1967:

> *'In every case, serum concentrations of vitamin B_{12} greater than 140 and 100 pg/ml persisted after hydroxocobalamin and cyanocobalamin-zinc tannate for twice as long as after cyanoco-balamin'.*[3]

(Note 'twice', not 'three times'.) But:

> *'However, differences between patients were very great, such that the entire trial with the three drugs was completed in 11 months in one case but lasted more than 4 years in another. Variation between patients makes it impossible to anticipate the duration of effect of a single injection of one of these drugs in any patient.'*[4]

In other words, the research showed what most sufferers of pernicious anaemia already know – that the one-size-fits-all rule for treatment is unsustainable because different patients have different treatment needs when it comes to the frequency of their injections.

And there's more:

> *'Following injections of cyanocobalamin and hydroxocobalamin most of the excretion occurred in the first 24 hours; with hydrox-ocobalamin the excretion was less than with cyanocobalamin'.*[5]

In other words, within 24 hours of having an injection 'most' of the injected B_{12} had disappeared in the patients' urine, whether the injection was of hydroxocobalamin or cyanocobalamin. True, the excretion of hydroxocobalamin was 'less' than of cyanocobalamin, but the question remains: can the body retain the remaining hydroxocobalamin for a full two months longer than it can B_{12} in the form of cyanocobalamin, especially when *most* of the injection disappears within a day? If the number of telephone calls, online forum topics, letters received and telephone callbacks made by the Pernicious Anaemia Society's nurse are indicative of anything, it is that hydroxocobalamin doesn't last very much longer than cyanocobalamin..

The guideline (and it should be just that – a guideline) that doctors follow when prescribing B_{12} in the UK is set out in the *British National Formulary*, or *BNF*.[ii] In the 1960s, the *BNF* stated that patients were to be given an injection of cyanocobalamin every two to three weeks. Then, when hydroxocobalamin became the replacement therapy of choice, the *BNF* said it should be given every two months, until the 1980s, when it was changed to 'every two to three months'. By the mid 1980s the *BNF* was stating that the injection should be given every three months. Interestingly, the duration of treatment was changed from 'for life' to 'usually for life' in the early 1980s. Whilst some doctors will deviate from the guidelines, others stick rigidly to what the *BNF* states. It is difficult to determine how many doctors do deviate from the guidelines because patients whose doctors *will* allow more frequent injections are unlikely to join the Pernicious Anaemia Society; their treatment is tailored

---

ii The *British National Formulary* or *BNF* is a British medical and pharmaceutical reference book that provides medical professionals with information on prescribing medicines including dosage and side effects. It is published by the Royal Pharmaceutical Society and the British Medical Association and distributed free to all practising NHS doctors in the UK. (The NHS picks up the tab.) Two new editions are published every year.

to their need. Certainly the vast majority of members of the Society, and therefore patients who I come into contact with, are unable to get a treatment regime based on their individual requirements.

In countries where cyanocobalamin is used, the injection is usually given every month. Table 8.1 shows information I have compiled (and am still compiling) about the type of B_{12} and the frequency of the treatment for individual countries.

Table 8.1 Standard treatment for pernicious anaemia provided in different countries ('OTC' stands for 'over the counter'.)

Country	Prescription or OTC	Treatment	Frequency
Australia	Prescription and OTC	Hydroxocobalamin	Two-three monthly Two monthly with neurological involvement
Canada	Prescription and OTC	Cyanocobalamin	Monthly
Finland	Prescription Prescription Prescription and OTC	Hydroxocobalamin Cyanocobalamin Cyanocobalamin tablets	Two-three monthly Two-four monthly 1-4 mg/day
France	Prescription and OTC	Cyanocobalamin	Monthly
Germany	Prescription and OTC	Hydroxocobalamin	
Ireland	Prescription	Hydroxocobalamin	Three monthly
Japan	OTC	Methylcobalamin	On demand
Netherlands	Prescription only	Hydroxocobalamin	Three monthly
Spain	Prescription and OTC	Cyanocobalamin	Monthly
United States	Prescription and OTC	Cyanocobalamin Hydroxocobalamin	Monthly
United Kingdom	Prescription only	Hydroxocobalamin Cyanocobalamin lozenges	Three monthly

Cyanocobalamin is the most widely used form of B_{12}. It does, however, have disadvantages for some patients. One study found smokers excreted 35% more B_{12} than non-smokers[6] and this was because tobacco smoke contains cyanide, which the body needs to get rid of; it is as cyanocobalamin in urine that the cyanide is eliminated so that smokers risk excreting the 'good' cyanide that is at the core of the cyanocobalamin along with the 'bad' cyanide found in tobacco smoke. In other words, smokers risk throwing the baby out with the bathwater.[7] This indicates that cyanoco-balamin may be actively excreted, rather than being retained as a source of B_{12} in people with elevated cyanide levels.

Others who may have problems using cyanocobalamin are those at risk of developing Leber's optic atrophy (which is he-reditary) as it can cause optic nerve damage. If you live in the UK and are sourcing B_{12} in the form of cyanocobalamin from mainland Europe (as the Table shows, this form of B_{12} is available over the counter in pharmacies in most of mainland Europe) it is important that you tell your doctor, especially if you know of any family history of Leber's optic atrophy. Even if you do not have such a family history, you should always tell your doctor if you are using any form of B_{12} other than that which has been prescribed, although I'm aware that many patients are nervous about discussing this with their doctor, fearing that he or she will stop writing out prescriptions for B_{12}.

Methylcobalamin is not licensed for use in the UK or North America, but it is widely available from doctors who register with a company that manufactures it in Texas. It can also be bought easily in the Far East in supermarkets, where different brands compete for market share. It is a 'purer' form of B_{12}, being closer to the form in which the body uses the vitamin: the body converts cyanocobalamin into hydroxocobalamin and then into methyl-cobalamin – the active form of B_{12} – before methylcobalamin mutates into adenosylcobalamin.[8] Adenosylcobalamin is ıstable and is not used to treat pernicious anaemia, but methylcobalamin is – where patients can get it.

Some doctors provide B_{12} infusions using methylcobalamin, where the patient is connected to a drip that slowly saturates every part of his or her body with this pure form of B_{12}. The patient, once saturated, can then give him or herself little subcutaneous injections to keep the level of B_{12} high. This is the regime I follow and it has meant that I can manage my condition better. I doubt whether I would have been able to write this book if I was on a three-monthly intramuscular injection of hydroxocobalamin. Again, you should discuss this alternative treatment with your doctor before receiving such an infusion and you should allow only a qualified and registered doctor to treat you in this way.

Consequences of one-size-fits-all treatment

There are two main consequences of the way pernicious anaemia is currently treated in the UK and some other countries. Firstly, allowing patients access to the vitamin that keeps them alive only via a doctor's prescription, in accordance with a rigid schedule, means that many thousands of patients are living lives that are anything but full. Just a short amount of time spent reading the online forum of the Pernicious Anaemia Society's website will show that patients' requests to their doctors for more frequent injections are routinely refused. This leads to patients often experiencing a return of their symptoms after just a few weeks, with all of the consequences that brings. They become lethargic, start forgetting things, start to underperform in the workplace and, if they have lost their jobs, will sit at home counting the days and weeks until they can get another injection. If the Pernicious Anaemia Society has achieved anything, it is to have shown that people need different treatment regimes centred on their *individual* needs.

Secondly, if a doctor refuses to depart from the *British National Formulary*'s guidelines despite clear evidence that symptoms have

Figure 8.1 PA Society Questionnaire – Chart showing the frequency with which respondents receive injections of vitamin B$_{12}$ (courtesy of the Pernicious Anaemia Society)

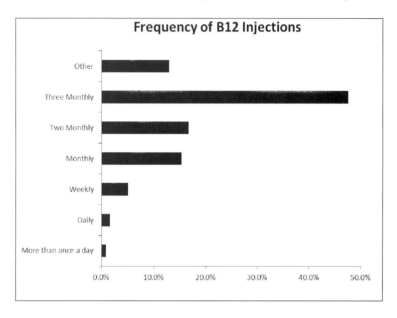

returned, the patient will feel frustrated and this often leads to a breakdown in the patient/doctor relationship. The number of wasted doctor appointments taken up with patients asking for, and being refused, more frequent injections can only be imagined; likewise the economic cost of taking time off work and travelling to the doctor's surgery for such futile visits. What members tell the Society is that this usually occurs many, many times before the patient either gives up or seeks an alternative source of injections.

When the Pernicious Anaemia Society first moved into a small office in 2007, the opening ceremony was conducted by the MP for Bridgend, Madeleine Moon. There was a handful of guests at the event and when Madeleine asked about the main problem for sufferers she was told it was the lack of adequate treatment for the majority of the members. One of the members present related his experience, which would be laughable if it didn't have such serious consequences. This is what he said:

> *'I am the manager of a care home for the elderly. My symptoms all came back a month after I had the injection and I went to my doctor twice asking for another injection, which I was refused. A week before my three months were up I booked an appointment with the practice nurse and turned up at the appointed time on a Friday. I remember that there was a sign on the door to her room requesting that patients remove their jackets and roll up their sleeves prior to being called into the nurse's room. I supposed that this was to save time. When I was in the room, with my sleeves dutifully rolled up, the nurse looked at her records and told me it was too soon for my injection as it had only been two months, three weeks and five days. She said I would have to come back on Monday. I was astounded. I told her that Monday was a public holiday and she just said I would have to make the appointment for the Tuesday instead. How stupid is that?'*

It's very stupid and unfortunately not uncommon. Doctors and nurses will often make the most outlandish statements as to why a patient cannot have more frequent injections. Here are a few that have been sent to me:

> *'Your liver will collapse.'*

> *'You'll start internal bleeding.'*

> *'The problem is that the more B_{12} you have, the more you will want; it's like heroin.' (A Practice Manager to a patient.)*

> *'Some people get high on too much B_{12}.'*

> *'You'll develop nerve problems if you have too much B_{12}.'*

> *'Your blood will thicken.'*

All of the above are, of course, nonsense. There is absolutely no evidence that a person can have too much B_{12} in his/her blood. Any excess is simply excreted in the patient's urine. This is because B_{12} is water soluble and so is completely harmless. Vitamin B_{12} can only do good.

The need for scientific evidence and new research

So why are doctors so against allowing their patients to receive treatment to correct B_{12} deficiency according to their need? Well, I think the answer is because doctors are scientists and there is no scientific research whatsoever that supports the notion that different people suffering from pernicious anaemia need different amounts of replacement therapy. Indeed, I've just given a reason why more frequent injections would, logically, do no good – any surplus is passed out of the patient's body in urine. What would be the point of sanctioning more frequent injections when the patient will simply excrete any surplus?

Once the patient has started with replacement therapy injections, any blood test used to determine the B_{12} status of his or her blood will almost inevitably show a normal or higher than normal level of B_{12} in the blood, even three months after the injection was given. This would support the argument that an injection every three months is an adequate treatment regime. If the serum B_{12} level is healthy then surely the patient can't need more frequent injections? Could it be that he or she is *imagining* the need for an earlier injection? Unfortunately, that is what most medical professionals believe – that the patient is imagining the return of the symptoms and that he or she does not need an earlier injection. However, the fact remains that the demand for more frequent injections is the single most common issue that concerns member of the Pernicious Anaemia Society.

Something is wrong with the current treatment and it badly needs investigating. It's a bit like cricket balls swinging in damp conditions: science hasn't been able to explain the phenomenon, but it certainly happens. (There has probably been much more research into cricket balls swinging than there has been into why different patients with pernicious anaemia need individual treatment regimes.)

The British National Formulary *and further consequences of a rigid treatment regime*

As described in footnote ii, the *BNF* provides information to medical professionals relating to the prescription of drugs in the UK. It is a reference work that is often consulted by doctors when writing prescriptions. Along with lots of other information, it states the frequency with which drugs should be administered. Here's what the current 62nd edition, published in September 2011, advises for B$_{12}$:

> 'By intramuscular injection, pernicious anaemia and other mac-
> rocytic anaemias without neurological involvement, initially 1
> mg 3 times a week for 2 weeks, then 1 mg every 3 months.'[9]

However, where there is neurological involvement this changes to:

> 'Pernicious anaemia and other macrocytic anaemias with neuro-
> logical involvement, initially 1 mg on alternate days until no
> further improvement, *then 1 mg every 3 months.*'[iv]

Now, what constitutes 'neurological involvement'? I would say that 'the fogs' – that sensation that nothing is clear, everything is confusing – memory loss and the inability to think of the name of everyday objects coupled with irrational behaviour and

iv My emphasis.

mood swings are all symptoms of neurological involvement and that numbness and balance problems are not the only neurological issues. And I'm not on my own in defining neurological involvement so. Dr Joseph Chandy is a GP in a busy practice in the North East of England. He has been aware of the consequences of B_{12} deficiency and how it affects the nervous system for 40 years. This is his interpretation of the *BNF* guideline:

> *'I consider "neurological involvement" to include problems with the peripheral nervous system such as pins and needles, numbness, tremor, foot drop, nerve and muscle pain (neuropathy, myopathy) and early signs of paralysis of limbs (sub-acute combined degeneration). But as well as the problems affecting the peripheral nervous system there are neurological problems with the central nervous system that include "fogs", cognitive decline, memory impairment resulting in dementia/Alzheimer's disease, loss of balance (ataxia), non-epileptic seizures, facial palsy, early Parkinson's-like presentation and MS-like [multiple sclerosis-like] presentation.'*

Dr Chandy is not alone among GPs in interpreting the *BNF* guidelines on 'neurological involvement' in this way, but it has to be said that it is a minority of GPs that do so.

So, what happens when a patient needs more frequent injections and is denied them by his or her doctor? People in the UK, North America, and Australia, where the ampoules of the injection are available only on prescription, source them elsewhere and inject themselves, or get a family member or friend to do so without the knowledge or consent of their doctor. Many patients in the UK simply travel to mainland Europe and buy ampoules of cyanocobalamin from pharmacists there. Those from North America, Australia and New Zealand, and other countries where the ampoules are available only on prescription, source the injections from the internet, whether or not they are reputable and reliable sources. Last week I bought some on eBay, even though it is against eBay's policy on medicines, which reads:

'Any substance or item that requires a prescription from, or the supervision of, a licensed practitioner (such as a doctor, dentist, optometrist, optician, pharmacist or veterinarian) to dispense isn't allowed on eBay.

'Some over-the-counter (OTC) products are allowed, as long as their listings neither mention nor compare them to prescription drugs. Worldwide shipping should not be offered on these items as it's impossible to verify whether it is legal for sale in every country. Similarly, please understand that items authorised for sale in other countries aren't necessarily authorised for sale in the United Kingdom.'

The problem is, of course, that in some countries the injections are available over the counter and in others only via prescription. When I queried the seller as to whether or not the B_{12} was in the form of injections or tablets he replied, 'Either – you know eBay's policy.' He might as well have added a smiley wink. I paid £10 for 10 ampoules, which arrived two days later. The ampoules were probably from Belarus.

The Pernicious Anaemia Society does not condone or encourage patients to buy injectable B_{12} from the internet. In fact, the Society advises strongly against doing so. And the Society, and I, suggest that, if the patient is going to go down the road of buying injectable B_{12} from sources other than their prescription, then he or she should *always* discuss this with their GP. They should also receive instructions as to how to inject safely and use sharps bins (for disposing of needles) and pre-injection wipes. At the time of writing I know that there are a great many members of the Pernicious Anaemia Society who have found alternative sources of B_{12} and are injecting themselves without any training, employing the same needle a number of times, without using pre-injection wipes and using empty jam jars as sharps bins. This has to be wrong and needs to be addressed urgently.

Health inequality

Over and above people who simply cannot afford to supplement their standard treatment, there are three groups of patients who are unable to source more frequent injections. Young children with either infant pernicious anaemia or juvenile pernicious anaemia do not usually request more frequent injections, but members of their families often report that there is a change in the behaviour of the child at the time of their next injection or a few weeks after they have received an injection. Bizarrely, every time the Society has received requests for information about a particular child it has always been the child's grandmother who has telephoned. The grandmothers all point out the same problems – that a few weeks after the child has received his injection (we've never had to deal with a young girl) the boy won't get out of bed and refuses to go to school. Sometimes, and I along with many other sufferers of pernicious anaemia will empathise with this, the child refuses to participate in class or group activities in the afternoons. Sometimes educational psychologists become involved and, when the child's doctor assures the psychologist that the child is receiving perfectly adequate treatment for his pernicious anaemia, unfortunately the psychologist will diagnose the child as having behavioural problems. That child will then carry that label all through his school life. These problems might easily be solved by giving the child more frequent injections.

The second group of patients who will not have access to more frequent treatment are the elderly, who may not be aware of how to access more frequent treatment. Community nurses are usually the professionals who provide the injections to these often vulnerable adults, and any community nurse will tell you that many of his or her patients know when their injection is due. There is a sinister side to the way in which the elderly are treated. Every week the Society gets at least one telephone call from either an elderly patient or an elderly patient's family or friend who is concerned that the patient has had his or her injections stopped 'because you no longer need them'. The member of the Society who is the manager of a care home and who related his experience of being told his injection couldn't be given because he was asking for it two days early is also able to bear witness to what amounts to abuse of elderly patients with pernicious anaemia. He told a meeting of the Society at Christmas 2010:

'One day, the nurse called and told three of my residents that they no longer needed injections. I had to go to the surgery and demand an interview with the doctor who had ordered the injections stopped. He reluctantly reinstated them. Luckily, as I have pernicious anaemia, I knew the consequences of the injections being stopped.'

One lady, who is 92, had been injecting herself every month for 40 years. When she went to the surgery to ask for a prescription for the ampoules she was refused. She telephoned the office and it was a very tearful telephone call. Thankfully her injections were reinstated after I had spoken to the community nurse, who then consulted with the patient's doctor.

The Society became aware of this problem of treatment being stopped only gradually, but, after presenting the evidence to the relevant authorities, the Medical Director of the National Health Service in Wales wrote to all doctors informing them that any GP who was identified as stopping B_{12} injections for elderly patients would be severely dealt with. We, as a Society, have had no further reports of Welsh patients being told they no longer need injections, but we still get them from members in the rest of the UK. One recent email stated that the patient's GP had told her that the government had written to all GPs stating that the B_{12} injections don't work in people over 65 years of age. Why are medical professionals telling elderly patients that they no longer need injections? I honestly don't know. All that I do know for certain is that it happens. One day I had three such reports before 10 o'clock.

The third group of people with pernicious anaemia who will not be able to access more frequent injections are to be found in the prison population. I spoke with the brother of one elderly man who was serving a prison term and who had asked the prison doctor for more frequent injections. 'My brother told me that it would be easier to get hold of heroin than get more frequent injections of B_{12},' he told me on the telephone.

Alternative B_{12} replacement therapies

What do Simon Cowell, Justin Bieber, Madonna, Lindsay Lohan, Gerri Halliwell and Robbie Williams all have in common? They are all keen recipients of injections of vitamin B_{12} that help them cope with the pressures of stardom or enhance their performances. Turner Prize-winning artist Tracy Emin has even complained that the injections only last two weeks.[10] It is unknown whether they source the injections from their GPs and whether or not they get them on prescription or from some other source. That they get them at all, without anyone taking blood samples or analysing symptoms, and get them on demand, is in direct contrast to the experiences of a great many members of the Pernicious Anaemia Society, whose pleadings for more frequent injections are usually rejected by their GPs.

Here's what journalist Chris Heath wrote after being granted an interview with Simon Cowell in a feature in the *Daily Telegraph Magazine* on 5th November 2011.

'Each week, Cowell has an intravenous drip with B_{12}, magnesium, vitamin C and, he says, "something for your liver"...

'Sometimes he has it done in the office, sometimes at home. Before the needle goes in, Cowell's arm is frozen with a spray so that it doesn't hurt. "Even when I'm having a viewing session with producers," he says, "she just sticks a needle in me and we carry on doing whatever we are doing." He is connected to the IV for around half an hour. "When you have it done, it's an incredibly warm feeling," he testifies. "You feel all the vitamins going through you; it's indescribable but very calming, and then it gives you energy for a good few days afterwards."

'The procedure was recommended to him two or three years ago by Danni Minogue, a former X Factor *judge, and through Cowell its popularity has been spreading. "Everyone I've recommended it to, they've absolutely loved it," he says. His IV woman often visits the studio when he's filming. "It sounds odd, but when you have it, it is fantastic… One girl came down and actually had two orgasms during the treatment." '11*

I've heard from lots of people who have benefited from B$_{12}$ infusions, but that's the first time I've heard of anyone getting sexual pleasure from it.

B$_{12}$ infusions are just one of the alternative treatment regimes that are available but are not used by the NHS in the UK or in many other countries. People who suffer from pernicious anaemia are unable to change their diets or swallow pills to correct the deficiency. However, a wide range of B$_{12}$ products has developed that by-pass the need for injections. They work by entering the blood stream via membranes in different parts of the body: the skin (intradermal), under the tongue (sub-lingual) or in the nose (nasal). This is the same way nicotine, for example, may enter the bloodstream: in pipe-smokers, it crosses into the blood through the mucous membrane that sits under the tongue; there is another such membrane in the nose (which is why snuff-takers sniff ground tobacco up their noses); and for those who want to give up smoking, nicotine patches allow nicotine to enter the bloodstream via the skin. Many patients buy these B_{12} supplements from internet companies and use them to top up their three-monthly or monthly treatments – just a short trawl of the web will give you some idea of the size of this market. They are relatively expensive and not all patients report any improvement, yet others rely on them to give them a quality of life that they would not have if they relied solely on the prescribed treatment regime.

The most amazing thing about all of these different treatments is that no government agency has tested their efficacy. There has been some preliminary research conducted into the efficacy of nasal sprays, but it hasn't been published. Zeena Nackerdien, a South African biochemist diagnosed with pernicious anaemia, and Derek Enlander, an Irish physician specialising in chronic fatigue syndrome, studied the effectiveness of methylcobalamin spray in rectifying B_{12} deficiency on 13 patients. Their preliminary findings suggest that the nasal spray worked well in their small group of patients. Table 8.2 shows the serum B_{12} levels of the patients before and after they had used the spray.

Table 8.2 Serum B_{12} levels measured in pg/ml in individuals before and after using the nasal spray (Nackerdien & Enlander)

Treatment:							
Before	667	439	720	818	744	525	536
After	1420	1360	2000	1833	2000	1844	2000
Patient	1	2	3	4	5	6	7

Treatment:						
Before	355	744	688	1200	622	734
After	877	1402	1520	2000	1482	1700
Patient	8	9	10	11	12	13

It is such a pity that these researchers didn't have the funding to follow the research through and experiment with a bigger cohort. Considering the high cost of administering injections,[v] it is hard to believe that none of the alternative methods has been examined to see if they might be of equal benefit to injections. Imagine the amount of nurse time that could be freed up. Such research, however, has the additional challenge that simply assessing the level of B_{12} achieved in patients' blood will not alone show the efficacy of any treatment. We know that just because a person has higher levels of B_{12} in his or her blood than a normal healthy person, it doesn't mean that the symptoms of B_{12} deficiency disappear. Something must be happening at cell level and these alternative, unevaluated preparations may hold the key.

It is not known how many patients are receiving supplementary treatments without their doctor's knowledge but it is fair to say that all over the world people are injecting, sniffing, spraying, sucking and dissolving all manner of B_{12} preparations – and that number is growing. The true figure will never be known but it is likely to be millions worldwide. To some extent, primary care doctors have lost control of their patients' treatment, which is another reason why somebody should start investigating why some patients need more frequent treatments than others. This would hopefully alleviate some of the worst consequences of inadequately treated pernicious anaemia, which we will now examine in the next chapter.

---

v It's not the cost of the ampoule of B_{12} but the cost in nurse time which is estimated to be £10. No government agency has considered teaching patients to self-inject using methylcobalamin, which can be administered subcutaneously by the patient and does not have to be injected into a muscle, which is how cyanocobalamin and hydroxocobalamin have to be delivered.

References

1   *The Anemias*. Indianapolis, Indiana, USA: Eli Lilly and Company, 1938.

2   Vidal-Alaball J, Butler CC, Cannings-John R, et al. Oral vitamin B12 versus intramuscular vitamin B12 for vitamin B12 deficiency. *Cochrane Database Systematic Review: The Cochrane Collaboration*, 2005; 20(3): CD004655.

3   Tudhope GR, Swan HT, Spray GH. Patient variation in pernicious anaemia, as shown in a clinical trial of cyanocobalamin, hydroxo-cobalamin and cyanocobalamin–zinc tannate. *British Journal of Haematology* 1967; 13(2): 216–228.

4   Ibid.

5   Ibid.

6   Food and Nutrition Board, Institute of Medicine. *Dietary Reference Intakes for Thiamin, Riboflavin, Niacin, Vitamin B6, Folate, Vitamin B12, Pantothenic Acid, Biotin, and Choline*. Washington, DC: National Academy Press; 2000.

7   Forsyth JC, Mueller PD, Becker CE, Osterloh J, Benowitz NL, Rumack BH, Hall AH. Hydroxocobalamin as a cyanide antidote: safety, efficacy and pharmacokinetics in heavily smoking normal volunteers. *Journal of Toxicology and Clinical Toxicology* 1993; 31(2): 277-294.

8   James A. Neubrander, MD, USAAA 2007 International Conference: Methyl-B12: Doing It Right! Methylcobalamin Update.

9   *British National Formulary*, 62nd Edition. London, UK: Royal Pharmaceutical Society & The British Medical Association. 2011: www.bnf.org

10   'Help! Get me a shot'. *Sunday Times*, 24th June 2007.
     The truth about vitamin shots. *Marie Clair*, 5th December 2007.

11   The *Daily Telegraph Magazine,* 5th November 2011.

Chapter 9

Neurological problems and vitamin B_{12} deficiency

Pernicious anaemia is a serious medical condition that has been largely ignored by the medical profession for many years, almost certainly because it is regarded as a problem for which a solution has been found. However, as chapters 1 to 8 have shown, there are serious issues still around diagnosis and treatment; the condition urgently needs to be revisited and a robust and reliable diagnostic test developed. Similarly there needs to be a review of how pernicious anaemia is treated, with an emphasis on the needs of the individual patient and not on dubious rigid instructions.

Left undiagnosed, vitamin B_{12} deficiency causes damage to the nervous system that affects the ability of nerve cells in the brain and spinal cord to communicate with each other effectively. Nerve cells communicate by sending electrical signals, called 'action potentials', down long fibres, called 'axons', which are covered by an insulating fatty substance – the 'myelin sheath' (see Figure 9.1). From the 14th week of pregnancy, the fetus starts to build this insulating layer around its developing nerves. Research has shown its main purpose is to speed up the impulses that travel along the nerves. This is a great simplification of what happens, but sufficient to understand the importance of vitamin B_{12} in this chapter. If you are interested, there are many websites where you can find more detail – that's my way of saying it's a complicated subject.

Figure 9.1 A neuron (nerve cell) showing the myelin sheath

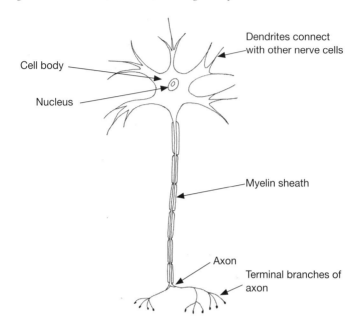

The myelin sheath was discovered by one the 19th century's most prolific medical men – the German, Rudolph Virchow. Virchow is regarded as 'the father of modern pathology' and has no fewer than 15 medical terms named after him, including 'Virchow's cell theory' that states that all living cells are the product of previously divided cells.[i] He lived until he was 80, this longevity being due in no small part to his having rejected an invitation to a duel by Bismarck, whose policy on military spending he opposed.

The important point here is that the myelin sheath is essential for nerve cells to send impulses effectively and a lack of vitamin

---

i There is some controversy about whether Virchow plagiarised the work of Robert Remak regarding this. Certainly it caused the two scientists to fall out over Virchow's claims.

B_{12} causes the myelin sheath to degenerate, leading to 'sub-acute combined degeneration of the cord secondary to pernicious anaemia'. This leaves the sufferer with varying degrees of numbness, balance and mobility problems, and cognitive impairment. 'Sub-acute' means neither acute (short term) nor chronic (long term). (Why doctors cannot make up their minds if the nerve damage is short term or long term is a mystery.) 'Combined' means that both the dorsal and lateral columns of the spinal cord are damaged, the myelin sheath surrounding the columns having degenerated. 'Degeneration' means just that: that the nerves have 'withered'; 'of the cord' refers to the spinal cord; and 'secondary' means this degeneration has been caused by a primary condition, in this case the patient's pernicious anaemia.

Degeneration of the myelin sheath is also the root cause of multiple sclerosis. So similar are the symptoms of sub-acute combined degeneration (SACD) of the cord caused by pernicious anaemia and multiple sclerosis that many members of the Pernicious Anaemia Society who have developed neurological problems have originally been suspected of having multiple sclerosis, and have been investigated for it. (Interestingly, though, only three respondents to the Society's survey had actually been diagnosed with multiple sclerosis before being correctly diagnosed with SACD.) It appears B_{12} deficiency is also sometimes coincident with multiple sclerosis. To quote a 1992 paper in the journal *Neuroimmunology*:

> 'It is useful to know that multiple sclerosis (MS) is occasionally associated with vitamin B_{12} deficiency. Recent studies have shown an increased risk of macrocytosis [enlarged distorted blood cells – see page 69], low serum and/or CSF[ii] vitamin

---

ii CSF stands for cerebrospinal fluid – the fluid that surrounds the brain, protecting it by acting as a cushion. Examining the CSF can identify diseases such as MS and meningitis. The fluid is extracted from the patient by lumbar puncture, sometimes known as a 'spinal tap'.

B_{12} *levels, raised plasma homocysteine and raised unsaturated R-binder capacity in MS. The aetiology [cause] of the vitamin B_{12} deficiency in MS is often uncertain and a disorder of vitamin B_{12} binding or transport is suspected. The nature of the association between vitamin B_{12} deficiency and MS is unclear but is likely to be more than coincidental. There is a remarkable similarity in the epidemiology [who in the population has a condition] of MS and pernicious anaemia. Vitamin B_{12} deficiency should always be looked for in MS. The deficiency may aggravate MS or impair recovery. There is evidence that vitamin B_{12} is important for myelin synthesis and integrity but further basic studies are required'.*[1]

It is claimed that B_{12} in the form of methylcobalamin promotes the re-myelination of affected nerves and can be used to treat peripheral neuropathies.[2] It is not licensed for use in the UK, Europe or North America, though it is widely and readily available from some doctors who know of its reputed value in repairing nerve damage, perhaps by repairing damage to the myelin sheath. I have been unable to find any reputable evidence to support these claims that methylcobalamin can repair or regenerate neurological damage other than in the information leaflet included in one brand of injections that is available in supermarkets in the Far East.[3] Most advertisements for methylcobalamin tablets or drops talk of 'neuron health' and 'brain health' but even Wikipedia fails to offer any evidence to support these claims. There are many references to methylcobalamin preventing or delaying Alzheimer's disease, but only one really important study supports these claims, as I will describe.

In September 2010, the results of a research programme that investigated brain shrinkage caught the imagination of the world. Scientists at the Oxford Project to Investigate Memory and Ageing (OPTIMA) had identified 168 elderly people experiencing levels of mental decline known as 'mild cognitive impairment'. Mild cognitive impairment leads to memory lapses and difficulty finding the right words to describe things. (Sounds familiar?) These symptoms can be the precursor to Alzheimer's disease. For two years, half of the 168 volunteers were given a daily tablet containing folic acid, B_6[iii] and B_{12} at doses way above the recommended daily requirement. The other half of the group were given a placebo.[iv] In a normal human being over the age of 60, the brain shrinks by 0.5% every year. People unfortunate enough to have mild cognitive impairment experience brain shrinkage of 2.5% annually. MRI[v] scans were used before and after the experiment to measure any shrinkage. At the end of the trial, the brains of those patients who were given the high dosage B vitamins were found to have experienced brain shrinkage between 30% and 50% *less* than those who were given the placebo, meaning that in some cases the patients were experiencing a normal rate of brain shrinkage.[4] Why did these B vitamins have this effect? Well, it seems that the vitamins lowered the level of homocysteine in the participants' blood. High concentrations of homocysteine are believed to be a cause of brain shrinkage that can lead to Alzheimer's disease. Now, with the Western world facing an ageing crisis, as more and more people live longer, with the consequent increase in age-related diseases, including brain shrinkage and Alzheimer's disease, wouldn't it make sense to screen the general population for B_{12} deficiency in middle age? I am unaware of any plans to introduce any such screening in the near future.

iii Also known as pyridoxine (PD).

iv The placebo in this case was a tablet that contained nothing that could have any health effect. Placebos are used in scientific experiments so that patients do not know whether they are receiving the active treatment or not, thereby ruling out any imagined benefit of taking the medication being tested.

v Magnetic Resonance Imaging – a type of medical imaging using powerful magnets.

As we saw in chapter 8, some doctors provide methylcobalamin infusions that slowly saturate every part of the patient's body with this 'pure' form of B_{12}. The patient, once saturated, can then give him or herself little subcutaneous injections to keep the level of B_{12} high. As I said in chapter 8, this is what I have had performed and it has changed my life. I've never had a 'fog' day since. As I also said, it is important you discuss this alternative treatment with your doctor before receiving this infusion and you should allow only a qualified and registered doctor to treat you in this way.

Somewhat amazingly, B_{12} in the form of methylcobalamin is also used to treat autism. To quote Dr James Neubrander:

'In my practice, 94% of children have been found to respond to Methyl-B_{12} therapy. Executive function is improved in 90% of children – things like awareness, cognition, appropriateness, eye contact when called, and "just being more like a normal kid." Speech and language is improved in 80% of children – all phases including spontaneous language, more complex sentences, increased vocabulary, etc. Socialization and emotion is improved in 70% of the children – initiation and interactive play, understanding and feeling emotions, possibly for the first time or to a much more normal degree, etc.'[5]

Patients diagnosed with subacute combined degeneration of the cord (SACD) secondary to pernicious anaemia will have outwardly visible symptoms, but to varying degrees. Many will experience numbness in their hands or feet or both. Some will have serious walking difficulties and balance problems. The Pernicious Anaemia Society calls these 'the shoulder bumps' as the patient will often bump against walls. Ascending stairs is usually not a problem whereas descending them is. The patient may have developed severe vertigo and will almost certainly have cognitive impairment, which means his/her intellect will be affected to varying degrees. Patients can and do have to use a wheelchair or other walking aids in the worst cases. In the UK, patients who have been diagnosed with SACD are usually registered as disabled and are eligible for a wide range of benefits to help them live as normal a life as possible. Apart from some patients responding well to methylcobalamin, the neurological damage will be permanent. In the worst cases, patients are left fighting their disability, which will have a profound impact on their everyday lives. One such person is a teenager from Ontario in Canada. Here's his story as written by himself on the Pernicious Anaemia Society's forum:

'Hi, my name is Joshua John Luckasavitch (nickname JJ). I am 13 years old. I have been asked to write this letter on how I got sick. Well here it goes. I have always had food allergies and asthma all my life. But in November of 2006 I got pneumonia and I was off school until January of 2007. I tried to go back to school after the Christmas break since I was feeling better but I only lasted a couple of hours. All of a sudden I didn't feel good so I asked my teacher if I could phone my mom to come and get me. My teacher told me to go to the office and phone home so I did. My mom met me and I just crossed Trulls Road and collapsed. My legs just gave out and I couldn't get up. From Trulls Road to my house it isn't far (about a 5-minute walk) but it took my mom about an hour to get me home. When we got home my mom phoned for backup for her daycare kids (she runs a nursery) and took me to the urgent care in Courtice and they sent me to the Oshawa hospital and they took a lot of tests. Even blood was taken. My skin was yellow (which the hospital said was jaundice). Which scared me because I heard the doctor tell my mom it could mean something is wrong with my liver. After about six hours at the hospital and all the tests the doctor there said he wanted me to go see a paediatrician so my mom asked if we could go to the same one that my sister is seeing for* *her headaches and he also was the one at the hospital when I was born. So they said yes so he gave my mom a referral. We went to the paediatrician and he took more tests and he thought it might be my liver so he sent me to a liver specialist at the Centenary hospital in Pickering. She also took more tests and she told my mom and dad that she was sending us to a friend of hers that is a liver specialist at Sick Kids Hospital in Toronto because she thought a liver biopsy was needed. So by now it was already February and I was getting worse. I was more yellow and I could hardly walk meaning I needed my mom and dad to hold on to me to help me walk since I was so weak and my legs were like jelly and I could hardly feel them. So we went to Sick Kids and met this doctor and he did major tests and by the end of the day this doctor thought I had a disease called Wilson's, which all I know about is that there is too much copper in your body and that it is rare and very serious. They decided to do the biopsy on my liver. The first appointment was cancelled by the hospital which was in March. So they finally did the liver biopsy at the end of March or beginning of April. The biopsy went good so we had to wait for the results. I was getting weaker and I felt really sick and so tired. My mom kept phoning the Doctor's office where the biopsy was done but they never returned her calls to let us know about the results of the biopsy or anything. So meanwhile I could feel like I was getting worse and we were still waiting for some kind of results so it is like July now so finally she took me in to see my paediatrician in Oshawa here and told him no one was phoning back with any results. So he was keeping a close eye on me and doing more blood tests. At this point I was worse, even the whites of my eyes were yellow now. I also couldn't keep food in me much. All I did was sleep.*

'My mom and dad rented a walker for me to help me walk. One weekend while at my trailer I was real sick and my urine didn't look good so my mom and dad know this lady at the

campgrounds and went to get her opinion and she said it didn't sound right so she drove my mom and me to Port Hope Urgent Care and they took a urine sample and asked for the results to be sent to my doctor back home. This lady's name is Donna and she is real nice. I think she helped me get into the hospital by getting me to get a urine sample done because finally the liver specialist phoned and said more tests had to be done and that they wanted a MRI done and that someone would phone my parents with a date and time. Now it is end of July and I finally get a date for the MRI because after my pediatrician called the liver doctor there seemed to be a cancellation. Then my mom got a call from the liver doctor saying he wanted to see me. On August 9th 2007 there had been a cancellation. By now I could not walk or even write or print plus I was having problems with my short term memory. We got to Sick Kids on the 9th of August and as soon as he saw me he said he was admitting me into the hospital to do further testing [because] the diseases they had thought I had had been ruled out. The next day they started doing all kinds of tests and there were so many doctors and interns. The same day they found out I was vitamin B_{12} deficient and low in all my other vitamins so they started me on vitamin B_{12} injections daily and I started feeling better but my liver count was still high so they continued to do more tests and I was told I had a long way to go. I was in Sick Kids for two weeks and was seen by so many doctors and had so many tests done that I just wanted to go home. Then about two weeks after I got home from the hospital the pediatrician from Sick Kids who is real nice phoned my mom and told us that some of the test results came back and that I have pernicious anaemia – (SACDSC) secondary to PA. I have nerve damage but I won't know how much until a year and a half from now. I need a laptop to type my assignments for school since I can't write or print no more plus I need programs for my laptop to help me. Plus I can't focus for long and I easily get frustrated *when doing things. I am being home schooled since I can't go to school. I get tired real easy and I need lots of breaks when I am doing my school work since I can't concentrate for a long period of time.*

'*I got a laptop donated to me since the school board didn't want to get one for me. So I have been going to Sick Kids Hospital every month getting checked out and getting blood tests and X-rays done. I have been in a lot of pain lately in my back so they ended up doing a bone density test and found out I have osteoporosis in my back and multi-fractures from my 10th vertebrae to my 4th so they are talking about doing a bone biopsy but so far it hasn't been booked yet. I am taking two vitamin B_{12} injections a week and vitamin B_{12} Methylcobalamin Quick Dissolve Sublingual tablets on the days that I don't get my injections. I have noticed I have more energy and can do more things than I could do before.*

'*About the beginning of June of this year the doctor decided to try to replace one of my injections a week with a vitamin B_{12} tablet, but within two days after not getting that one injection I felt more tired and my legs got weaker than they were before and I started throwing up again. When my mom had seen the way I was she put me back on the injection like before and within a week I was back with more energy and I could keep food down again. I feel a lot better with the second injection a week. I have been able to go to school one day a week for a couple of hours and then I come home and rest but it feels so good being able to go to school even for a couple of hours to see my friends.*

'*I did have a setback a couple of weeks ago. Some of my vitamin levels came down, especially my vitamin D, so I am on these D drops which I take one drop a day. With this I have noticed a difference. I have been able to go swimming twice so far at my trailer park with my friends. Plus I have been able to walk without my walker a little way as long as someone is with me in case I get tired and need a rest.*

'This week I got to go to school a couple of times and spend time with my friends and help prepare for my grade 8 graduation. Yesterday I went to school for my rehearsal and then got my report card which was really good (lowest mark 71 and my highest was 85) then all the grades from kindergarten to grade 7 lined up in the hallways and they had to clap all of us grade 8s out of the school which made me feel real good mainly because I did all this without my walker. I then went home and rested because last night I had my graduation and got my diploma which means I will be in grade 9 in September of this year. I also did all this without using my walker but by 11 pm I was ready to come home because I was sore and tired. I went straight to bed.

'I learned one huge thing – that my principal and my family were right because a year ago I was so sick and was dying and I was told not to give up which was hard not to because this year was so hard with me being so sick and fighting to get better. And my Grandpa who was also my godfather died in January of this year of cancer and then my best friend's dad died in March of this year, which even made it harder not to give up. But with all this I also made a promise to my Grandpa before he died that I wouldn't give up so I didn't. Then last night I also remembered what my principal Debbie Ford said a while ago to the whole entire school that I have had a rough year and through everything I was like her hero of the school because I never gave up and it proves to the whole school and to everybody that you can still stay caught up in your school work and pass your grade.

'So I have realized that I have met one of my goals. I wanted to walk into my class at school without my walker and to graduate grade 8 without my walker and go to graduation not using my walker and guess what, I did it all. And I finally feel good about

myself because I believe if you have faith anything can happen, which for me came true. I met my goal for this year. Now I start working on my next goal and that is to be able to go to high school gradually until I make it the whole day. This is it for now except to thank everyone for not giving up on me.

Joshua

PS I will get my mom to add to this when there is more to update.'

I travelled to Canada to meet with JJ. He walked to me without his walker. His mother told me he was determined to meet me standing on his own without any aid.

Because of the serious consequences of patients having a delayed diagnosis it is particularly important for the way in which pernicious anaemia is diagnosed and treated to be seriously examined and revised as soon as possible. At the time of writing, the UK's National Institute for Health and Clinical Excellence has posted eight questions about the way in which pernicious anaemia is diagnosed and treated in the hope that a researcher will pick up on the questions and propose a research programme to answer these. At last, it seems medical professionals are beginning to listen to patients' concerns. Given that there is some evidence that methylcobalamin carries many more benefits than the other synthetic forms of B_{12}, it is hard to explain why no robust investigation into its use has taken place. However, the issue is further complicated by some patients reporting that they respond better to either cyanocobalamin or hydroxocobalamin, and so the ideal solution would be to allow the patient a choice in his or her form of treatment. Patients with neurological damage should be treated with methylcobalamin as the evidence is that it helps promote re-myelination, which

·ld obviously benefit these patients. Until more research is
ı into this, it should be remembered that, according
sh *National Formulary,* if the patient has 'neurological

involvement' he or she should be getting a 1 mg injection[vi] *every other day* until there is no further improvement.

As Joshua's story illustrates, left untreated, vitamin B_{12} deficiency can have a profound effect on people's lives. Not only does it affect the patient but also the patient's family and friends, their careers and lifestyles. The economic implications are also enormous, not only for the individual and his or her family, but for the national economy as a whole.

References

1   Reynolds EH. Multiple sclerosis and vitamin B12 metabolism. *Neuroimmunology* 1992 ; 40(2-3): 225-230.

2   The following references are provided on the information sheet that is enclosed with the methylcobalamin vials manufactured by Eisai, which proudly boasts that the injections are used to treat peripheral neuropathies:

Ogawa T et al: *Vitamin* 1989; 63: 123.

Kameyama M et al: *Japanese Journal of Clinical and Experimental Medicine.* 1972; 49: 1967.

Marauyama S et al: *Japanese Journal of Clinical and Experimental Medicine.* 1989; 66: 995.

Inada M et al: *Nervous Systems and Methyl B12 (Kyowa kikaku tsuushin)* 1981; 23.

Nakazawa T er al: *Vitamin* 1970; 42: 193.

Nakazawa T et al: *Vitamin* 1970; 42: 275.

Takenaka T et al: *Vitamin* 1982; 2: 1759.

Ohnishi A et al: *Japanese Journal of Clinical Pharmacology & Therapeutics* 1987; 18: 387.

Watanabe T et al: *Journal of Neurological Science* 1994; 122: 140.

Saitoh T et al: *Nervous Systems and Methyl B12 (Kyowa kikaku tsuushin)* 1981; 75.

Yamazaki K et al: *Neuroscience Letters* 1974; 170: 195.

Yagihashi S et al: *Japanese Journal of Clinical Pharmacology and Therapeutics* 1988; 19: 437.

Nakagawa T et al: *Nervous Systems and Methyl B12 (Kyowa kikaku tsuushin)* 1981; 54.

Yonezawa T et al: *Nervous Systems and Methyl B12 (Kyowa kikaku tsuushin)* 1981; 49.

vi Of hydroxocobalamin.

Shibuya T et al: *Nervous Systems and Methyl B12 (Kyowa kikaku tsuushin)* 1981; 134.

Sasaki H et al: *Pharmacology Biochemistry and Behaviour* 1992; 43: 635.

3   Ibid. [what details does this refer to?]

4   Smith AD, Smith SM, de Jager CA, et al. Homocysteine-lowering by B vitamins slows the rate of accelerated brain atrophy in mild cognitive impairment: a randomized controlled trial. *PLoS ONE* 5(9): e12244. doi:10.1371/journal.pone.0012244

5   Neubrander J. Methyl-B12: a treatment for ASD with methylation issues. http://www.tacanow.org/family-resources/methyl-b12-a-treatment-for-asd-with-methylation-issues/

Is B$_{12}$ a performance-enhancing drug?

One of the strangest telephone calls that I have taken happened on a Friday morning in late 2009. I answered the 'phone with the usual 'Good morning. Pernicious Anaemia Society'. A gruff voice went straight to the point. 'Is vitamin B$_{12}$ a performance-enhancing drug?'

I hesitated.

'I suppose it depends on what a performance-enhancing drug is,' was my unhelpful reply. I asked the caller who he was. I can't recall his name and I didn't write it down, probably because I was so shocked by the nature of the call, but I *do* remember he said he was from UK Athletics, the UK's national governing body for athletics. I asked if one of his athletes had been using B$_{12}$ and he didn't reply directly but asked again if it was a performance-enhancing drug.

'It's a vitamin,' I told him.

'But does it enhance performance?' I thought for a moment and then told him that I knew it was given to racehorses. He thanked me and the conversation ended. I don't know the story behind the call, nor do I know if athletes take B$_{12}$ to enhance their performance or if there was any investigation. Perhaps this issue will resurface sometime in the future.

Chapter 10

The consequences of pernicious anaemia

Pernicious anaemia has varying effects on people's lives. Some patients manage perfectly well on the standard replacement therapy injection given every three months and carry on living normally. Others adopt a variety of coping strategies to manage their condition. Others, less fortunate, have to make life-changing decisions in order to cope with their illness.

It isn't known why some people are only mildly inconvenienced by pernicious anaemia whilst others struggle to cope with even the most mundane of everyday tasks. It was only with the advent of the Pernicious Anaemia Society that patients who had for many years been told that they must be imagining their symptoms because their B_{12} deficiency had been corrected found others in the same position as themselves. The Society's online forum and regular meetings have meant that patients who had previously felt isolated and alone now have others who empathise with them. One thing that is certain is that a great many patients with pernicious anaemia are still symptomatic to varying degrees even after replacement therapy has been established.

The reasons for this have not been explained and, because there is no robust scientific research to support the complaints of the patients, medical professionals usually attribute their ongoing symptoms to their imaginations. Patients who make repeated visits to their doctors complaining that they are still experiencing the continual tiredness, irritability and exhaustion are regularly labelled as hypochondriacs. That patients are still symptomatic after receiving loading doses of B_{12} and then regular replacement therapy injections could be due to the length of time they suffered before the B_{12} deficiency was identified and treated. It could be that the longer a patient waits for a diagnosis and treatment, the more likely he or she is to carry on experiencing the symptoms of the condition. Nobody knows because nobody has investigated this. It is much easier to tell patients that they are imagining their problems and suggest they might benefit from some anti-depressants.

There is no cure for pernicious anaemia, and, as far as I'm aware, nobody is looking for one. Whilst the level of B_{12} in a patient's blood can be brought back to normal, the symptoms often never completely disappear. And these symptoms not only have an impact on the everyday life of the patient; they also affect the patient's family, social life and contribution in the work place. More broadly, they also have an impact on the economy. The Pernicious Anaemia Society is in a unique position in being made aware of how pernicious anaemia affects patients' lives, and the lives of their families and friends. It campaigns to get medical professionals to understand that injections of B_{12} might keep patients alive, but they don't always relieve the symptoms. Here I will try to highlight these ongoing effects, but please understand that the degree to which the condition affects lives depends on the severity of the symptoms in each individual.

Social issues

The extent to which the patient's condition affects his or her life will depend on exactly what symptoms are experienced and the severity of those symptoms. The first thing to realise therefore is that every case will be different.

The first major impact that pernicious anaemia has on social life concerns the patient's family. Mix together lethargy, exhaustion, irritability, mood swings and the need for quiet and calm, and you have all of the ingredients for family problems. The condition may lead merely to the patient having to go to bed earlier than he or she used to; it can lead to severe and irreparable relationship breakdown. The worst scenario I have come across was when a mother was investigated by social services because she was having to sleep in the afternoons and could often not wake in time to collect her children from school. Thankfully, with the intervention of the children's grandmother, the family stayed together.

The social side of family life will often have to alter, with evenings spent out with family members being a thing of the past. Then there are sexual health issues, especially if the patient has sub-acute combined degeneration of the cord (see page 155). It affects the patient's libido, patience and rationality. And unless the family are able to understand this, the patient may be ostracised by other family members and feel increasingly isolated and alone. It is very difficult for people who do not have pernicious anaemia to understand how the condition may alter personality and lifestyle. But there is another problem that makes this misunderstanding worse. If the patient re-visits his or her doctor asking for something to help relieve the symptoms, the doctor will usually suggest that, because the patient's B_{12} blood level is normal, or above normal, then the patient must be imagining the symptoms. The family members will usually believe the doctor and they too will then label the patient a hypochondriac or as suffering from depression. And there is still another sting in the tail. The patient *will* become depressed, simply because the quality of his or her life is so poor.

In 2011 the Pernicious Anaemia Society produced a documentary that featured interviews with its members and with medical professionals. Over 600 members bought a copy and showed it to their families. The result was that many members posted on the online forum, telephoned or wrote to the Society stating that for the first time their family members had understood what they were experiencing and that they were not imagining the symptoms. The DVD has gone some way to solving the problem of patients having unsympathetic families, but it hasn't stopped people with pernicious anaemia from feeling isolated. I regularly take calls from patients who have been given the Society's telephone number by their doctors and, when I empathise with them and talk openly about the problems that they face, invariably they end the conversation with, 'You are the first person who has understood what I am going through,' or words along those lines. I remember the first time the Society hosted a coffee morning for local members, I had trouble getting them to leave after five hours of talking to other sufferers. No matter how sympathetic family members are, only those who have had the same symptoms are able to fully understand how pernicious anaemia affects the everyday life of sufferers.

The impact that pernicious anaemia has on a patient's wider social life will vary considerably. Personally, I cannot imagine going out in the evenings. Like thousands of other sufferers, my day ends at around 6 pm and just the thought of socialising in the evening fills me with dread. I have to say again that some patients will have no problem whatsoever in attending events held in the evening and leading a life just the same as if they did not have pernicious anaemia. Others will be able to attend evening events but cannot get up in the mornings – it all comes down to the individual.

There are two social-life issues to be aware of. Firstly, if the patient fights the tiredness, fatigue and exhaustion and attempts to do all the things he or she used to do before developing the condition, then he or she will lose. I have come across this many times. The patient gets diagnosed and assumes that the past few weeks, months or years are now behind him or her and that a

Figure 10.1 PA Society Questionnaire – Chart showing how respondents rated the medical care they had received in relation to the diagnosis and treatment of pernicious anaemia (courtesy of the Pernicious Anaemia Society)

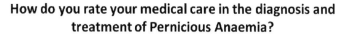

How do you rate your medical care in the diagnosis and treatment of Pernicious Anaemia?

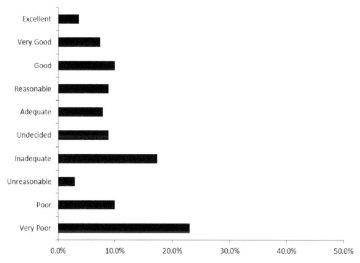

normal, full-on lifestyle can be led. Usually this doesn't happen and the patient will 'pay the price' for going against what his or her body is telling him/her. Earlier this year I was asked to be Best Man to an old friend who was getting married. When I was asked I immediately thought about what time of day the ceremony would take place; as we all know, it is usually early in the day so I replied that I would happily carry out my duties to the best of my ability and that I was honoured to be asked. My heart sank when I was told the wedding would take place at 3 pm. I stayed out until 9 pm and it took me a week to recover.

Secondly, and perhaps more importantly, the patient should, but doesn't always, manage his or her condition by making small, medium or large lifestyle changes. It doesn't mean that the patient cannot have, or expect to have, a social life comparable to that of people without pernicious anaemia; rather, by making allowances, changing the way he or she lives and lowering expectations, he or she can have a social life of sorts. It's all to do with managing the condition. I don't know when I last went out for dinner, but I often meet people for lunch. I can't remember when I last went to the cinema in the evening, but know from experience that cinemas tend to be very quiet in the afternoons. Any meetings of the Trustees of the Pernicious Anaemia Society always take place in the late mornings as do any meetings of members of the Society. Christmas celebrations revolve around our annual Christmas lunch – a very refined affair. However, it isn't always that easy. Those who have demanding jobs, or are responsible for looking after children or relatives, do not have the option of just switching off when they feel like doing so. I genuinely sympathise with such patients. Life is a daily struggle not only to carry out his or her duties, but also to fight against the symptoms of pernicious anaemia. No wonder patients with such onerous demands on them, and who are expected to go three months between injections, have suicidal thoughts – 23.6% of those who undertook the Society's survey.

Juvenile pernicious anaemia

The impact that pernicious anaemia has on the social life of teenagers and young adults is especially sad. Whereas I had a very full early life, playing in bands, DJ'ing, walking mountains, playing tennis, chasing (and sometimes catching) girls and women, it grieves me to take telephone calls and have face-to-face conversations with young people whose personal lives are so affected by pernicious anaemia. It isn't just that the constant tiredness and lethargy mean any nightlife activities come with a heavy price. It's also very difficult for young people with pernicious anaemia to form long-term relationships because they will not want to go out in the evenings and need to sleep for 12 hours every night.

Then there are children who have pernicious anaemia. The youngest member of the Pernicious Anaemia Society was just 18 months when her mother joined on her behalf; her brother was the second youngest at four years old. It is impossible to know just how many children have pernicious anaemia, but the grandmothers who have contacted the Society all convey the same message – that the school doesn't understand the condition and that the children affected display all of the symptoms of the disease a few weeks after their injections. Two of the young sufferers known to the Society had major dental surgery with nitrous oxide used as the anaesthetic. Nitrous oxide destroys B_{12}.

One other aspect of juvenile or infant pernicious anaemia also has to be noted. We saw in chapter 7 how there is a strong genetic link for the condition. Parents who have pernicious anaemia should always bear this in mind and be aware that, contrary to what is commonly believed, pernicious anaemia is not just a disease suffered by old women.

Pernicious anaemia seriously affects family life. Unfortunately it often leads to the break-up of relationships; this seems to be caused not by one party not tolerating the behavioural changes in their partner, but by the partner not understanding why the changes have taken place. This is exacerbated by medical professionals assuring patients that once they start having replacement therapy injections all should be well. The partner therefore believes that the incessant tiredness, lethargy and mood changes are not a consequence of the pernicious anaemia. Hopefully, this book will explain why the patient acts as she or he does and go some way to preserving relationships.

Denny is a 39-year-old solicitor (name changed). She has studied hard all her life and has finally become a partner in one of the top 50 law firms in the UK. Denny arranged to meet me in Hyde Park in London. She was displaying all the signs of B_{12} deficiency – fighting to find words, repeating herself, seeming distant. She was encountering all kinds of problems at work.

'I'm making all kinds of silly mistakes,' she told me. 'I'm missing things that I would never in a million years have missed before. And the worst thing is, I am in danger of being found out by my colleagues. I really don't know what to do.'

Clare works for the Welsh Assembly. She was diagnosed four years ago with classic pernicious anaemia. 'I'm okay until about two o'clock and then I just stare at my computer screen and wait for five o'clock,' she told me.

Anthony is a police constable; or rather, he was a police constable. 'I just couldn't cope with the shift patterns. Nobody understood anything about the illness and I lost my career.'

'I just couldn't cope,' Janice, a former school teacher, told me. 'I struggled for three years, but would come home from work, open the front door and go straight up the stairs to my bed. I was existing rather than living.'

These are just a small selection of stories that illustrate how pernicious anaemia affects the careers and jobs of thousands, maybe millions, of patients throughout the world. One of the saddest aspects of running the Pernicious Anaemia Society is hearing the pleas for advice on how to cope with workplace issues and how to keep doing the job the patient loves. It's the most difficult advice to give because I know, from personal experience, that the patient is often trying to carry on with a career that he or she is no longer capable of.

There are two issues surrounding workplace problems caused by pernicious anaemia. Firstly, as with domestic issues, it is believed almost universally that once the patient receives replacement therapy, then the symptoms will disappear. And the fact that for some patients this is exactly what does happen confuses the issue further. The employer believes this and so does the employee, because his or her doctor has told him/her so. All are wrong. Again, the degree to which the patient still experiences the symptoms of pernicious anaemia will differ from individual to individual. This gets worse if the employee finds him/herself involved in an employment tribunal; most medical professionals, called to give evidence, will state quite categorically that the patient should now be completely free of the symptoms as the B_{12} deficiency has been rectified.

Secondly, employers are not obliged to make any concessions for patients with pernicious anaemia because the seriousness of the symptoms is not generally recognised. If employers seek outside advice – usually from a medical professional – they will be told that symptoms should resolve, and this is made worse if there are other employees in the same organisation who have pernicious anaemia and who can manage perfectly well with their day-to-day employment. Pernicious anaemia is simply not regarded as a serious disease – it is thought of as a type of anaemia that is 'cured' by injections of a vitamin. We are back to the question that has plagued this book. Why do some people respond perfectly well to the replacement therapy injections while others remain symptomatic? In the past year I have been asked to write a letter to trades union representatives on three occasions. I had been contacted because the union was representing one of its members at an employment tribunal. I was able to give the patient view of dealing with workplace issues, but on no occasion have I been told of the outcome.

Economic issues

There are millions of people in the world suffering from pernicious anaemia and who are still symptomatic even after their B_{12} deficiency has been corrected. These patients are at a loss to understand why, though they should be symptom-free, they are not. They struggle in the workplace, often underperforming and making costly mistakes. They make repeated visits to their doctors and are often prescribed expensive drugs. The cost to the economy cannot be measured because no research has been done in this area. Dr Hugo Minney has been studying the effects of B_{12} deficiency for many years. He has calculated that the cost of erroneously prescribed drugs, handed out in an effort to treat patients who still have the symptoms of B_{12} deficiency even though they are receiving B_{12} injections, is a staggering £854 million in the UK every year. That's just the cost of unneeded prescriptions. That doesn't take into consideration the many millions of pounds spent by the NHS in the UK on doctor visits and the accompanying time off work. The total cost to the UK economy alone probably runs into billions of pounds every year.

As we saw in the previous chapter, left undiagnosed and untreated, pernicious anaemia leads to serious, irreversible nerve damage caused by the lack of B_{12} which is needed to maintain the myelin sheath that coats nerve fibres. This can lead to permanent disability and patients relying on carers to help them perform everyday tasks. I will leave it to you to try to estimate the cost to the patient, the patient's family, society and the economy for not diagnosing a vitamin deficiency soon enough.

The future

I hope that this book will act as a catalyst to reawaken interest in pernicious anaemia. That has been a key intention in writing it – that it will help individual patients and their families to understand better the condition and feel less isolated. Reading this book, it may have seemed at times that I am highly critical of medical professionals. I am not, but I am critical of any medical professional who, after reading this book, is still of the opinion that the way in which vitamin B_{12} deficiency in general, and pernicious anaemia in particular, is diagnosed and treated is perfectly acceptable. There are some serious issues that need to be dealt with and some even bigger scientific questions that need to be answered.

Thankfully, there are still doctors who are prepared to depart from conventional guidelines and treat patients according to their individual needs. These doctors are the kind that listen to patients – I mean actively listen and treat their patients accordingly. Unfortunately, they are far too few in number, which makes treatment for pernicious anaemia something of a lottery. And this has gone on far too long.

If I was to compile a wish list to solve all of the many issues surrounding the diagnosis and treatment of pernicious anaemia, then it would look something like this:

1. Immediately raising the threshold used to determine B_{12} deficiency to 300 pmol/l as advocated by Professor Smith and Professor Refsum. Maybe it should be raised even higher to around the 500 pmol/l as Sally Pacholok and Jeffery Stuart advise. What is certain is that the current level of around 140 pmol/l is far too low.

2. Evaluate the effectiveness of the 'active B_{12}' test in identifying B_{12} deficiency and its usefulness in monitoring B_{12} levels to ensure that no further deficiency occurs.

3. Evaluate and make available where appropriate different, more economical methods of treatment based on the individual patient's choice and needs. This would include the option for the patient to receive hydroxocobalamin injections delivered by a health professional.

4. Make the medical profession and the general public aware that patients with pernicious anaemia experience the symptoms of their condition to varying degrees even after B_{12} replacement therapy has begun. Why this is so needs to be investigated.

5. Make screening for B_{12} deficiency a routine practice – including screening young people.

6. Find a cure for pernicious anaemia so that hopefully, in the future, the condition can be eliminated and not just treated.

7. Evaluate the effectiveness of the new emerging treatments and make these available to whoever needs them.

I have had my life changed by pernicious anaemia and have dedicated the last eight years to providing information, help and support not only to patients, but also to their families and friends. I have not done this alone but have had the support and encouragement of a great many people, including my family, fellow trustees and the other marvellous volunteers who help run the Society. It's been a hard eight years but I remain hopeful that this book will go some way to attaining the wish-list seen above. I am realistic enough to understand that this will probably take a long time to achieve; it could be a very long time, but I am also confident that we will, eventually, get to where we want to be and achieve the vision of the Society, which is to live in:

'a world that understands the nature and consequences of pernicious anaemia and where there is easily accessible information, advice and support for sufferers and their families.'

And with the values of the Society in place:

'... respect for the right and dignity of our service users to choose their preferred treatment method that allows for a flexible and individually tailored regime that is focused on the individual needs of the patient in order that they can best manage their condition.'

With your help and support this is possible, though as one respected investigator has put it, 'To the stalwart little band of investigators of vitamin B_{12} there is comfort in knowing that the stream of important scientific problems will never end'.[1]

Reference

1   Beck WS. Cobalamin and the nervous system. *New England Journal of Medicine* 1988; 26: 1752-1754.

Appendix 1

The discovery of vitamins and their food sources

Year of discovery	Vitamin		Food source
1910	Vitamin B_1	(Thiamine)	Rice bran
1913	Vitamin A	(Retinol)	Cod liver oil
1920	Vitamin C	(Ascorbic acid)	Citrus and most fresh food
1920	Vitamin D	(Calciferol)	Cod liver oil
1920	Vitamin B_2	(Riboflavin)	Meat and eggs
1922	Vitamin E	(Tocpherol)	Wheat germ oil/Unrefined vegetable oils
1926	Vitamin B_{12}	(Cobalamins)	Liver/Eggs/Animal products
1929	Vitamin K_1	(Phylloquinone)	Green leafy vegetables
1931	Vitamin B_5	(Pantothenic acid)	Meat/Whole grains – Many foods
1931	Vitamin B_7	(Biotins)	Meat/Dairy products/Eggs
1934	Vitamin B_6	(Pyridoxine)	Meat/Dairy products
1936	Vitamin B_3	(Niacin)	Meat/Eggs/Grain
1941	Vitamin B_9	(Folic acid)	Leafy green vegetables

Appendix 2

Resources and further reading

Symptoms of pernicious anaemia

Everyone is different and sufferers of pernicious anaemia will experience the symptoms of the condition to varying degrees. Some patients will have all of the symptoms listed in the table below while others will recognize only a few. This table has been compiled over a number of years and shows what a wide range of symptoms there can be. There are two problems with this wide range. Firstly, many of the symptoms listed below are associated with other medical conditions. Secondly, because there are so many symptoms associated with pernicious anaemia it makes it difficult for doctors to identify the symptoms *specific* to the disease – thus making an early diagnosis even less certain.

For fuller descriptions of the symptoms listed, please refer to chapter 2.

Common general symptoms
- Shortness of breath – 'the sighs'
- Extreme fatigue
- Brain fog
  - o Poor concentration
  - o Short-term memory loss
  - o Confusion ('handbag in the fridge syndrome')
  - o Nominal aphasia (forgetting the names of objects)
- Unaccountable and sudden bouts of diarrhoea, often follow-

ing a spell of constipation
- Clumsiness/lack of coordination
- Brittle, flaky nails; dry skin anywhere on body
- Mood swings, 'tear jags', heightened emotions
- Sleep disturbance
  - o Even though patient is exhausted, is unable to sleep
  - o Waking up still tired, even after many hours' sleep

Neurological symptoms
- Balance problems
  - o Dizzy/faint
  - o 'shoulder bumps' – frequently bumping into or falling against walls
  - o General unsteadiness, especially when showering and dressing
  - o Inability to stand up with eyes closed or in the dark
  - o Vertigo – inability to cope with heights, linked to the need for a visual reference as compensation for damage to the brain's balance mechanism
- Numbness/tingling – especially in hands, arms, legs, feet
- Burning sensation in legs and feet – Grierson-Gopalan syndrome
- Tinnitus – ringing/screeching/howling in the ear or ears
- Neuropathic pain/fibromyalgia – often on only one side of the body
- Irritability/frustration/impatience; desire for isolation, quiet and peace; aversion to bright lights and crowded spaces

Skin problems
- Hair loss – can range from moderate to sever; premature greying of hair
- Psoriasis/eczema/acne
- Rosacea – reddening of the skin around the nose and cheeks
- Vitiligo – white patches that develop on the skin

Associated medical problems
- Poor digestion

- Arrhythmia – irregular, fast or slow heartbeat

Associated autoimmune conditions

- Rheumatoid arthritis
- Hypo- or hyper-thyroidism – almost exclusively among females
- Coeliac disease – sensitivity to wheat and/or wheat products
- Myasthenia gravis – weak muscles leading to problems swallowing, chewing and opening eye(s)
- Psoriatic arthritis

B_{12} deficiency test

The following questionnaire was devised by the Pernicious Anaemia Society to raise awareness among the general public that small, annoying, everyday sensations, if viewed alongside other similar sensations, can become part of a bigger picture that indicates B_{12} deficiency – that is, it is the sum of the symptoms that is significant rather than each symptom viewed individually. This test alerts anyone who completes it that he/she may be suffering from the effects of B_{12} deficiency whether or not that deficiency is caused by pernicious anaemia. Depending on how many boxes you tick, you will either be satisfied that you are not B_{12} deficient, or you will be enabled when you next visit your doctor's surgery to make him or her aware of your symptoms. If your score is very high, you should make an urgent appointment to see him/her.

Could you be B_{12} deficient? (reproduced with the permission of the Pernicious Anaemia Society)

Tick the boxes which correspond to your symptoms.

Strange tiredness	
'The fogs' – lack of clarity/difficulty in concentrating	
Breathlessness – 'The sighs' or 'The gulps'	
Sudden unaccountable bouts of diarrhoea	

Brittle nails	
Brittle nails *with ridges*	
Pins and needles – usually in your hands and feet	
Swollen and/or sore tongue	
Balance problems	
General unsteadiness	
Vertigo	
Burning legs or feet	
Tinnitus	
Irritability/anger/lacking patience	
Family history of B_{12} deficiency/pernicious anaemia	
Hair loss	
Dry skin (including scalp)	
Lack of concentration	
Memory loss	
Insomnia	
Premature greying of hair	
Psoriasis/eczema/acne	
Rosacea	
Arrhythmia	
Vitiligo	
Anaemia	
Infertility	
Dizziness	
Bleeding gums/mouth ulcers	
Loss of appetite/weight loss	
Neuropathic pain	
Numbness	
Depression/anxiety	
Confusion	
Blurred vision	

Note – this test is for information only and is NOT an aid to self-diagnosis. Your doctor is the best person to give you advice. This test is NOT a substitute for advice from your doctor.

© The Pernicious Anaemia Society – registered charity no. 1115195

Medicines that can interfere with vitamin B$_{12}$ absorption

A comprehensive list of commonly prescribed medicines that interfere with B$_{12}$ absorption can be found in *Could it be B$_{12}$? An Epidemic of Misdiagnosis* (see Further reading below). Particularly important to note are:

- Proton pump inhibitors – prescribed for heartburn and/or gastritis, ulcers, Helicobacter pylori infection and upper gastrointestinal bleeding. Examples: Prevacid, Prilosec, Protonix, Nexium, Adiphex, Omeprazole.
- H$_2$ blockers – also used to treat heartburn, gastritis and ulcers. Examples: Antac, Tagamet, Axid, Pepcid.
- Antacids – neutralise stomach acid. Examples: Alternagel, Maalox, MOM, Myulanta, Riopan, Tums.
- Biguanides – used to treat diabetes. Examples: Metformin, Glucophage, Riomet, Fortamet, Glumetza, Obimet, Dianben, Diabex, Diaformin, Glucovance.
- Potassium deficiency medicines – prescribed to treat potassium deficiency caused by kidney failure, congestive heart failure, cirrhosis of the liver or 'water pills'/ diuretics. Examples: K-Lor, K-Lyte, Lotrix, K-Dur, Micro-K, Slow-K, potassium chloride.
- Colchicine – used to treat gout
- Questran – used to lower cholesterol levels
- Neomycin – used to treat infections

- Para-aminosalicylic acid – used to treat tuberculosis
- Nitrous oxide – used in dental operations (also used as a recreational drug)
- Oral hormonal contraceptives (NB data about these are conflicting)

Support groups

Further advice and support can be found by contacting:

The Pernicious Anaemia Society
Level Four
Brackla House
Brackla Street
BRIDGEND
CF31 1BZ, UK
Tel: +44 (0)1656 769717
www.pernicious-anaemia-society.org

The Vitamin B_{12} Deficiency Group
www.b12d.org

Other forms of support can be found on the various B_{12} deficiency and pernicious anaemia pages on Facebook.

Sources of supplements

You should always consult your doctor before taking any supplements to your prescribed medication. Please note that the efficacy of the supplements listed below has not been evaluated in a scientific way.

If you are pregnant, nursing or taking any medications, consult your doctor before use. Discontinue use and consult your doctor if any adverse reactions occur.

Be aware that taking supplements will affect any blood tests that you undergo to determine the level of your serum B_{12}, and also remember that you will need good folate status (healthy levels of folic acid) for the B_{12} supplementation to work.

There are a host of bona fide companies selling B_{12}-related supplements in almost every country. Simply entering 'B_{12} supplements' into a search engine, will return a large number of sources of the vitamin. One company (yourhealthbasket) offers a 10% discount to members of the Pernicious Anaemia Society. Amazon and eBay both have a wide variety of B_{12} supplements, including skin patches and sublingual drops.

www.yourhealthbasket.co.uk
Unit 1, The Old Applestore
Chantry Farm
Chantry Lane
Boreham
CM3 3AN, UK
Tel: +44 (0)1245905505
Yourhealthbasket sells a wide range of B_{12} supplements including sub-lingual lozenges, nasal sprays and sub-lingual drops.

Betrinac
This new product has been developed based around 1 mg of B_{12} in cyanocobalamin form and also contains folic acid and N-acetylcysteine (NAC), which is an amino acid that increases levels of an important antioxidant, glutathione. Glutathione is the body's natural antioxidant defence. Many patients with pernicious anaemia find that taking NAC helps combat the continual tiredness that they experience.

In the UK, Betrinac can be contacted on 0800 689 9606.
Website: www.betrinac.com

Specialists

There are a number of doctors who provide a comprehensive range of treatments:

The British Society for Ecological Medicine is a society of qualified doctors who practise complementary medicine and who are aware of the importance of adequate B_{12} status. They can be contacted at:
Administrator
BSEM
c/o New Medicine Group
144 Harley St
London W1G 7LE, UK
Or via their website – www.ecomed.org.uk

Dr Manjeet Riar has helped a great many of the members of the Pernicious Anaemia Society and he conducts clinics in Bridgend, South Wales, and at Ashford in Kent. He can be contacted on +44 (0)1656 646815.

The Lytham St Anne's Clinic in the UK is attended by a medical doctor and provides infusions of methylcobalamin B_{12}. The web address is: www.b12treatment.co.uk

Further Reading

Until recently there was a dearth of written material on pernicious anaemia and B_{12} deficiency. This problem has been addressed by Sally Pacholok and Jeffery Stewart's *Could It Be B_{12}? An Epidemic of Misdiagnosis*. (Second edition, 2011, Quill Driver Books, California, ISBN 978-1-884995-69-9). This magnificent work pulls no punches and is a comprehensive overview of the problems caused by B_{12} deficiency being wrongly diagnosed and the consequences for healthcare.

Index

British National Formulary (BNF), 136, 139–140, 143–144, 164
burning sensation in legs/feet, 58

Cabot, Richard Clark, 98
Callendar, Sheila, 106
Canada
  daily B_{12} intake recommendations, 31
  PA treatment in, 137
carbon dioxide in blood, 25
career impact, 174–175
Castle, William B, 98
cereals *see* breakfast cereals
Chandy, Dr Joseph, 144
cheese, 35
children
  with autism, 158
  with PA, 88, 146, 172–175
chyme, 103, 104, 105
cobalamin see vitamin B_{12}
Cobalamin News, 17n
cobalt in soil, 39–41
coeliac disease, 61, 183
co-existing conditions, 58–62
cognitive impairment, 51–55, 144, 155, 158–159
  mild, 157
Cohn, Edwin, 100, 129
Combe, Dr James Scarth, 91, 92
confusion, 51–55, 143, 182
  see also fogs
consultant haematologist, author's experience, 10
co-ordination problems, 56–57, 182
coping strategies, 167
  author's story, 12
cost issues, 175–176
Could it be B_{12}?, 13, 77
Cowell, Simon, 148–149
cyanocobalamin, 23, 101, 136, 137, 138, 164
  non-prescription sources, 144–145

daily B_{12} intake recommendations, 31–35, 37
dairy products, 31, 37, 179
dental surgery and B_{12}, 173, 186
depression, 20, 49, 66, 67, 80, 96, 124, 169
  author's story, 4
diagnosis of B_{12} deficiency, 65–89, 120–121, 177
  author's story, 5–7
diagnosis of PA, 88, 111–126
diarrhoea, 58, 60, 181
diet
  healthy/balanced, 31
  vitamins and their deficiency in, 20–21
  see also food; nutrient
digestion, 104–106
duck egg, 34

eBay, B_{12} on, 144–145
economic impact, 175–176
egg, duck, 34
elderly
  mild cognitive impairment, 156–157
  PA treatment, 146–147
Emin, Tracy, 148
employment impact, 174–175
Enlander, Derek, 150
enterohepatic circulation of B_{12}, 27
enzymes, digestive, 104, 105
erythrocytes see red blood cells
Eschemoser, Albert, 101
European countries, PA treatment in, 137
evidence-based treatment of PA, need, 142–143

faeces (stools), B_{12} in, 106
family history of PA, 121–122
family life, impact of PA, 169–170
  child with PA, 173
fat-soluble vitamins, 22

Index